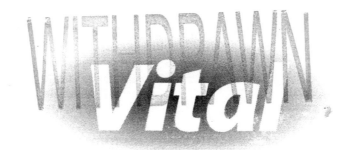

WITHDRAWN

Vital

DIABETES

*Your <u>essential</u> reference for the management
of diabetes in primary care*

Charles Fox BM, FRCP
*Consultant Physician with Special Interest in Diabetes,
Northampton General Hospital Trust*

and

Mary MacKinnon MMedSci, RGN
Diabetes Education Consultant, Sheffield

CLASS HEALTH · LONDON

Printing history
First published 1999, reprinted 2000
Second edition 2002, reprinted 2004
Third edition 2005, reprinted 2006
Fourth edition 2007
Monochrome edition 2009

The authors and publishers welcome feedback from the users of this book. Please contact the publishers.

Class Publishing, Barb House, Barb Mews, London W6 7PA, UK
Telephone: 020 7371 2119 / Fax: 020 7371 2878 [International +4420]
Email: post@class.co.uk

A CIP catalogue for this book is available from the British Library

ISBN 978 1 85959 227 4

10 9 8 7 6 5 4 3 2 1

Edited by Richenda Milton-Thompson

Designed and typeset by Martin Bristow

Printed and bound in Great Britain by Good News Press Ltd, Ongar, Essex

Contents

About the authors

Charles Fox BM, FRCP is a Consultant with Special Interest in Diabetes at Northampton General Hospital Trust, with over 30 years of experience. He is co-author of *Diabetes – the 'at your fingertips' guide*, the classic patient reference book which is about to be split into two editions, the first concentrating on type 1 diabetes, the other focusing on type 2. He also wrote *Diabetes in the Real World* (winner of the Richard Asher Award from the British Medical Association), on how to manage diabetes in general practice.

Mary MacKinnon MMedSci, RGN has nearly 30 years' experience of diabetes care in primary and specialist health care settings. She co-ordinated diabetes services in Sheffield for 10 years and set up diabetes education for nurses at the University of Sheffield.

She was a co-founder and Director of Education of Warwick Diabetes Care, the University of Warwick, and has contributed to diabetes development nationally and internationally.

Mary was the author of the first four editions of *Providing Diabetes Care in General Practice* and has been a pioneer in facilitating the extended role of nurses in diabetes care.

Comments on *Vital Diabetes* from readers

'Excellent book – good quick reference material for use within the clinical area.'

Julie Grindley, Practice Nursing Sister,
Audlem Medical Practice, Crewe

Dear Colleagues

Welcome to this new edition of *Vital Diabetes*

As the number of people diagnosed with type 2 diabetes continues to rise, diabetes care is changing. Nowhere is this more apparent than in primary care. So this practical book, aimed at those of you who work in general practice or the community, has been updated with your needs in mind.

Reflecting the prevalence of the two forms of diabetes among your patient population, this book focuses mainly on type 2 diabetes. The information it contains is designed to help you look after people who have this serious medical condition, as well as their near relatives (who often have such an important role to play in health care). Treatment of type 1 diabetes is also mentioned.

Presentation of the major studies on diabetes outcomes and care, along with recent policy documents such as the NSF and the GMS Contract, underpin the book. The text is divided into 14 distinct **chapters**, with topics clearly presented, and there is a detailed **contents list** to help you find your way around the book with ease. At the end of each topic, we have listed one or more **vital points** to give you essential information in just a few words.
The majority of chapters also contain sections on **patient and carer information**, which can be enlarged and photocopied for your patients.

You will find useful **appendices** and other information at the end of the book, including references, glossary, further reading and details of courses. We would welcome your comments or suggestions for improvements. You will find a **feedback form** on page 117.

We hope you will find this book helpful, time-saving and vital to your everyday clinical practice – and that, in using it, you will be able to provide an up-to-date and consistent standard and quality of health care for people with diabetes.

Charles Fox and Mary MacKinnon

Acknowledgements

We would like to thank Anne Kilvert, Consultant in Diabetes Medicine at Northampton General Hospital Trust, for her many important suggestions for improving the text and for the section on ASCOT; Maria Mousley, Consultant Podiatrist in Northampton, for her help with the foot care section; and our editor Richenda Milton-Thompson.

'Diabetes is an easy disease to treat badly.'
Professor Robert Tattersall

The impact of a diagnosis of diabetes is very powerful and affects all aspects of a person's life, either in general (eg the possibility of reduced life expectancy) or in particular (eg the need to lose weight and keep to a healthy diet).

Most people with newly diagnosed diabetes feel insecure. They are not sure about two important questions:

- Whether diabetes will interfere much with their lifestyle
- What they are expected to do about it

If they have type 2 diabetes, they may also worry about whether or not they have a serious disorder. (The smaller number of patients with type 1 diabetes are more likely to recognise this as serious.)

Badly treated diabetes means patients are:

- Not being consulted about their ideas about diabetes
- Ill-informed and unable to make choices about their own care
- Not being involved or taking the lead in their own diabetes care plan
- Not being the most valued and important member of their health care team
- Being told that they have 'mild diabetes' which could have been avoided
- Being unaware of the aim and possible consequences of their treatment
- Made to feel censured if ideal weight is not achieved or maintained
- Condemned for not achieving their target blood glucose level
- Made to feel guilty – treatment failure is all their fault
- Punished by the threat of insulin injections

■ Frightened at the prospect of insulin injections and the long-term complications of diabetes

The result of badly treated diabetes is a life filled with fear and guilt. Personal relationships and relationships with health carers may be severely compromised and even, occasionally, break down completely.

Badly treated diabetes does not provide care for individuals in the context of their cultural, psychological and social framework.

Well-treated diabetes involves patients:

■ Being competently assessed on diagnosis by a properly trained person

■ Being aware of research activity and new insights in diabetes

■ Taking the lead and being involved in their own (staged) diabetes care plan, wherever possible

■ Being able to make informed choices about their own care

■ Feeling valued and that they are the most important member of the health care team

■ Knowing that type 2 diabetes is not 'mild' but a serious and complex medical condition with associated long-term complications

■ Knowing about long-term complications, and how to reduce them

■ Understanding that diabetes cannot be cured, but that it is not their fault

■ Knowing that the underlying causes are insulin resistance and progressive beta-cell (β-cell) failure – and given explanation

■ Being informed that treatment for type 2 diabetes is often progressive and that insulin therapy is usually required sooner rather than later if optimum (agreed) blood glucose targets are not achieved

■ Knowing about the positive role of reduction in blood glucose and blood pressure levels in reducing the presence and severity of long-term complications

■ Understanding that reducing cholesterol with a tablet is important to reduce risk of heart failure and stroke

■ Feeling reassured, on diagnosis, that insulin injections are not to be feared – and given a practical demonstration (even if diet-only treatment is needed)

- Being aware of the risks and implications of medication and insulin therapy in the achievement of blood glucose and blood pressure (agreed) targets

- Having their cultural differences recognised and incorporated into their diabetes care plans, as far as possible

- Knowing that they are not alone; other people with diabetes can help

- Knowing what care to expect, who will provide it and how, and where to get it locally

- Understanding that most diabetes care is provided in the community and that secondary and tertiary services are involved, working with their general practice team

Well treated, the impact of type 2 diabetes will also be reduced if relatives and carers are involved. They should aim to know as much as the person with diabetes and be consulted in order to provide the necessary standard of support for the person concerned.

Well-treated diabetes involves caring for the person with sensitivity, taking into account their cultural concerns, psychological well-being, health beliefs and social structures in an individualised and thoughtful manner. The person with diabetes is central to care planning, and should be valued, well informed and empowered to make decisions about self-treatment and care.

VITAL POINTS

* Diabetes is a difficult disease, which can be well managed
* Value the person with diabetes (and those close to them)
* Enable them to make their own decisions

2 Insights into type 2 diabetes

There is continuing new evidence and insight into the management of type 2 diabetes. Five relevant studies have been completed and are summarised below. (Full references are all given on page 112.)

1 UNITED KINGDOM PROSPECTIVE DIABETES STUDY (UKPDS)

- UKPDS is still the largest clinical study of diabetes ever conducted
- It investigated the effect of intensive treatment of type 2 diabetes in reducing long-term complications
- It demonstrated that long-term complications are reduced with intensive therapy
- It showed that a reduction in HbA1c of 1% was associated with 14% fewer myocardial infarctions, 21% fewer deaths related to diabetes and 37% fewer microvascular complications
- It confirmed that type 2 diabetes is a serious and progressive disease, and NEVER 'mild'
- Up to 50% of people with type 2 diabetes were found to have long-term complications on diagnosis, emphasising the need for early detection and screening of those in high-risk groups
- There were valuable epidemiological findings, namely that there is no lower limit for reducing risk from blood glucose or blood pressure (ie the lower the better)
- Key treatment targets, reducing long-term complications in the study, relate to tight blood pressure and intensive blood glucose control

UKPDS Risk Engine

Most risk calculators for coronary heart disease are based on equations from the Framingham Heart Study, which tend to underestimate risks for people with diabetes (this study included relatively few diabetic subjects). The UKPDS Risk Engine, however:

- Is a type 2 diabetes specific risk calculator, based on 53,000 patient years of data from the UK Prospective Diabetes Study, which also provides an 'approximate margin of error' for each estimate
- Provides risk estimates and 95% confidence intervals, in individuals with type 2 diabetes not known to have heart disease, for:
  - Non-fatal and fatal coronary heart disease
  - Fatal coronary heart disease
  - Non-fatal and fatal stroke
  - Fatal stroke
- These can be calculated for any given duration of type 2 diabetes based on current age, sex, ethnicity, smoking status, presence or absence of atrial fibrillation and levels of HbA1c, systolic blood pressure, total cholesterol and HDL cholesterol

The UKPDS Risk Engine can be downloaded free from the website www.dtu.ox.ac.uk/ukpds. Click on Risk Engine in the left-hand column.

VITAL POINTS

* *Treatment targets (UKPDS) are:*
* *Blood pressure levels of < 130/80 mmHg*
* *HbA1c levels of < 7.0%*
* *Fasting blood glucose levels of 4–7 mmol/l*
* *Self-monitored blood glucose levels before meals of between 4 and 7 mmol/l*

2 PREVALENCE AND INCIDENCE OF TYPE 2 DIABETES IN THE UK (POOLE 1998)

- It is estimated that 1.53 million people are currently diagnosed with type 2 diabetes in the UK
- Another million may be undiagnosed
- Over 100,000 people are diagnosed with diabetes each year in the UK (one person every 5 minutes)

- The number of cases among men is significantly higher than among women
- This is a marked change from the position in the 1950s and 1960s, when cases among women were higher. The cause of this shift is unknown
- Factors contributing to the increase in diabetes include advancing age of the population, obesity and a sedentary lifestyle
- Groups at particularly high risk are those who are aged over 40 years, and who:
  - Are overweight
  - Are of Asian or Afro-Caribbean origin
  - Have a family history of diabetes
  - Have a prior history of gestational diabetes

VITAL POINTS

* *Ensure that people are aware of diabetes symptoms, lifestyle factors and serious complications*
* *Identify those at high risk*
* *Provide best possible care to prevent the onset of complications*

3 PRIMARY CARE DIABETES
– A NATIONAL SURVEY

- A national survey in England and Wales (Pierce *et al* 2000) aimed to describe the following:
  - The extent and organisation of general practice diabetes care
  - Primary care perceptions of support by secondary care
  - Cooperation with secondary care
  - Educational experience in diabetes of doctors and nurses in primary care
- The enquiry confirmed that the focus of diabetes care had shifted over the previous decade, the majority now being provided within general practice

- Practice nurses have become central to the delivery of good diabetes care

- There are significant geographical variations in the delivery of primary diabetes care

- One in five practices in England and Wales was surveyed, with a 70% response rate

Some results

- Median number of diabetes patients per practice is 110

- 75% of patients with diabetes are described as having most or all of their diabetes care in general practice

- 68% of practices had a special interest in diabetes

- 96% of practices had diabetes registers

- 87% of practices used their registers for call and recall

- 77% of practices had fully computerised registers

Key messages

- A large volume of diabetes care takes place in primary care

- Those providing it are very enthusiastic

- Nurses are important and the key to success

VITAL POINTS

* *Variations in primary diabetes care need exploring*
* *Education for GPs and nurses needs more development*

4 THE HEART PROTECTION STUDY (2003)

- This study was conducted under the auspices of the Medical Research Council and the British Heart Foundation

- Over 20,000 patients aged 40–80 years with cardiovascular risk factors were recruited into a study to investigate the effect of reducing cholesterol with a fixed dose of a statin (simvastatin 40 mg daily)

- Nearly 6,000 of the subjects had diabetes
- A well-designed study, which showed that reducing cholesterol in this way led to a 24% reduction in cardiovascular problems
- This finding was consistent, and not affected by age and gender, cholesterol level
- The relative risk reduction is remarkably constant but the absolute benefit clearly depends on the individual's baseline risk
- Serious side effects were very rare: with over 10,000 patients in each group:
  - Myopathy occurred in only ten patients in the simvastatin group and four in the placebo group
- The results of this trial have led to calls for diabetes treatment guidelines to be re-examined

More information about the results on this study can be found on the website (for details see page 114).

Complementary findings

- Another study, the CARDS Trial (2004) also found that cardiovascular problems were significantly reduced by the prescription of a statin (in this case, atorvastin) – the results being sufficiently conclusive to merit the study being stopped early
- CARDS is the first clinical trial specifically designed to investigate the effectiveness of cholesterol-lowering statin in people with type 2 diabetes who have no previous history of heart disease or stroke

VITAL POINTS

* *Lowering cholesterol by the prescription of statins results in a significantly reduced risk of cardiovascular problems*
* *Results have been confirmed by other studies (CARDS 2004)*
* *Findings are sufficiently dramatic to suggest a radical review of diabetes treatment guidelines is needed*

5 ASCOT (ANGLO-SCANDINAVIAN CARDIAC OUTCOMES TRIAL)

- This multicentre international study recruited over 19,000 patients with hypertension, but no previous or current coronary heart disease, to a two-armed trial of the effect of antihypertensive and lipid-lowering therapy on cardiovascular outcomes

- Approximately 4,500 subjects had type 2 diabetes

- The lipid-lowering arm (LLA) reported in 2003 and confirmed the findings of other cholesterol-lowering studies with a significant reduction in fatal and non-fatal stroke, coronary events and total cardiovascular events in patients with initial cholesterol < 6.5 mmol/l treated with atorvastatin 10 mg daily compared with placebo

- The blood pressure-lowering arm (BPLA) was stopped early because of a clear benefit to patients treated with a combination of amlodipine and perindopril compared with those taking atenolol and bendrofluazide. This study reported in 2005

- Although the primary endpoint of non-fatal myocardial infarction (including silent MI) and fatal coronary heart disease did not reach statistical significance, this was probably because the study was stopped early

- There were a number of positive secondary endpoints in favour of amlodipine/perindopril. These included cardiovascular mortality, non-fatal (excluding silent) myocardial infarction, fatal/non-fatal stroke and unstable angina. Post hoc analysis showed a reduction in revascularisation procedures in the amlodipine group

- Combined results from both arms of the trial showed:
  - Risk reduction for fatal myocardial infarction and non-fatal coronary heart disease was 48% for patients treated with amlodipine/perindopril/atorvastatin compared with those treated with atenolol/bendrofluazide/placebo
  - Risk reduction for fatal and non fatal stroke was 44% for those in the amlodipine/peridopril/atorvastatin arm

- New onset diabetes was reduced by 29% in the amlodipine/peridopril group. This could be due to withdrawal of bendrofluazide, a protective effect of perindopril or a combination of the two

The British Hypertension Society is reviewing its guidelines in the light of the results of ASCOT and other studies. It is likely that ACE inhibitors and calcium channel blockers will be recommended as first line treatment and that beta blockers will reserved for patients with ischaemic heart disease.

VITAL POINTS

* *The results of ASCOT and other studies are changing practice guidelines*
* *Care should be taken if beta blockers are withdrawn from therapy because of the risk of unmasking previously unrecognised heart disease*

3 National Service Frameworks and NICE

The National Service Framework for Diabetes was launched in December 2001, with the publication of the *Standards* document, followed 18 months later by the *Delivery Strategy* document.

STANDARDS

■ **Standard 1:** Prevention of type 2 diabetes
- ◆ The NHS will develop, implement and monitor strategies to reduce the risk of developing type 2 diabetes in the population as a whole, and to reduce the inequalities in the risk of developing type 2 diabetes

■ **Standard 2:** Identification of people with diabetes
- ◆ The NHS will develop, implement and monitor strategies to identify people who do not know they have diabetes

■ **Standard 3:** Empowering people with diabetes
- ◆ All children, young people and adults with diabetes will receive a service which encourages partnership in decision-making, supports them in managing their diabetes, and helps them to adopt and maintain a healthy lifestyle. This will be reflected in an agreed and shared care plan in an appropriate format and language. Where appropriate, parents and carers should be fully engaged in this process

■ **Standard 4:** Critical care of adults with diabetes
- ◆ All adults with diabetes will receive high-quality care throughout their lifetime, including support to optimise the control of their blood glucose, blood pressure and other risk factors for developing the complications of diabetes

■ **Standards 5 & 6:** Critical care of children and young people with diabetes
- ◆ All young people with diabetes will receive consistently high-quality care. With their families and others involved in their care, they will be supported to optimise the control of their blood glucose and their

physical, psychological, intellectual, educational and social development

- All young people with diabetes will experience a smooth transition of care from paediatric diabetes services to adult diabetes services, whether hospital or community-based, either directly or via a young people's clinic. The transition will be organised in partnership with each individual and at an age appropriate to and agreed with them

■ **Standard 7:** Management of diabetic emergencies

- The NHS will develop, implement and monitor agreed protocols for rapid and effective treatment of diabetic emergencies by appropriately trained health care professionals. Protocols will include the management of acute complications and procedures to minimise the risk of recurrence

■ **Standard 8:** Care of people with diabetes during admission to hospital

- All children, young people and adults with diabetes admitted to hospital, for whatever reason, will receive effective care of their diabetes. Wherever possible, they will continue to be involved in decisions concerning the management of their diabetes

■ **Standard 9:** Diabetes and pregnancy

- The NHS will develop, implement and monitor policies that seek to empower and support women with pre-existing diabetes and those who develop diabetes during pregnancy to optimise the outcomes of their pregnancy

■ **Standards 10, 11 & 12:** Detection and management of long-term complications

- All young people and adults with diabetes will receive regular surveillance for the long-term complications of diabetes
- The NHS will develop, implement and monitor agreed protocols and systems of care to ensure that all people who develop long-term complications of diabetes receive timely, appropriate and effective investigation and treatment to reduce their risk of disability and premature death
- All people with diabetes requiring multi-agency support will receive integrated health and social care

The service framework described in the *Delivery Strategy* should be used in conjunction with current and forthcoming guidelines and appraisals from the National Institute for Clinical Excellence (NICE). There are 6 sections:

- ■ **Section 1:** Introduction

- ■ **Section 2:** Building capacity
  - ◆ The 40-page implementation document asks for the setting up of diabetes networks to carry out the following roles: planning, delivery, leadership, information and monitoring. This should take place in the first year

- ■ **Section 3:** Delivering targets (3 years)
  - ◆ By 2006, a minimum of 80% of people with diabetes to be offered screening for the early detection (and treatment if needed) of diabetic retinopathy as part of a systematic programme that meets national standards, rising to 100% coverage of those at risk of retinopathy by end 2007
  - ◆ In primary care, update practice-based registers so that patients with CHD and diabetes continue to receive appropriate advice and treatment in line with NSF standards. By March 2006, ensure practice-based registers and systematic treatment regimens, including appropriate advice on diet, physical activity and smoking, also cover the majority of patients at high risk of CHD, particularly those with hypertension, diabetes and a body mass index (BMI) greater than 30 kg/m^2
  - ◆ The Delivery Strategy includes specific recommendations for improving care of people with diabetes: 'PCTs can also plan further care and interim review around a range of local options, such as timed review, problem solving visits, telephone review, direct access to blood pressure monitoring or HbA1c results, structured education and as part of structured cardiovascular care'
  - ◆ The recommendations for patient education that coincide with the aims of the DESMOND project (see page 48): 'advice and information about the importance of diet, physical activity and cessation of smoking to avoid the risk of developing the complications of diabetes'
  - ◆ 'Evidence has shown, however, that giving advice and information through group structured education programmes is one of the most effective ways of doing so. Good practice suggests that a structured

education programme is tailored to the individual, taking account of age, social circumstances, disability and ethnic, cultural and religious influences'

■ **Section 4:** Delivering Standards (10 years)

♦ The previous section focuses on Standard 3, and this section deals with the remaining 11 standards. These must be achieved by 2013 and the NSF recommends that the targets need to:

● be determined on the basis of local needs and service capacity

● be challenging

● be underpinned by information and workforce developments

● be costed and resourced

● have measurable outcomes

● be owned and agreed by the local health and diabetes communities

● demonstrate a clear trajectory to deliver all the standards by 2013

♦ The NSF highlights the importance of periods of transition (eg moving from school to university) as times when routine care may be more difficult

■ **Section 5:** Ensuring progress

♦ This section is concerned with monitoring progress of the NSF Diabetes project. It includes tools for Continuous Quality Improvement such as comparative benchmarking and HLPIs (High Level Performance Indicators)

■ **Section 6:** National support for local action

♦ The longest section in the document, detailing programmes designed to help local services implement the NSF, including the National Clinical Director for Diabetes, NICE and with patient and public involvement

THE NATIONAL INSTITUTE FOR HEALTH AND CLINICAL EXCELLENCE

The National Institute for Health and Clinical Excellence (NICE) is part of the NHS. It is the independent organisation responsible for providing national guidance on treatments and care for people using the NHS in England and Wales. NICE's guidance is intended for health care professionals, patients and their carers to help them make decisions about treatment and health care. NICE currently has eight documents (three Guidance documents and five Clinical Guidelines) that relate to type 2 diabetes.

Guidance documents

- Guidance on the use of insulin glargine:
  - ◆ Sensible, if cautious advice
- Guidance on the use of glitazones:
  - ◆ Positive about use of glitazones
  - ◆ Triple combination therapy is widely practised in the UK. However, the appraisal committee did not put forward a recommendation
- Guidance on the use of patient-education models
  - ◆ Recommends structured education by multidisciplinary teams
  - ◆ There is a shortage of experimental evidence to support the value of education

Clinical Guidelines

- Renal disease:
  - ◆ Distinguishes between low and high risk patients
  - ◆ Stresses the importance of measuring microalbuminuria and the value of ACE inhibitors in protecting the kidney
- Retinopathy:
  - ◆ Stresses the importance of controlling blood glucose and blood pressure to reduce eye problems
  - ◆ Recommends annual screening by retinal photography
- Blood glucose:
  - ◆ Recommends a target HbA1c of 6.5–7.5%, with the lower target for patients with a high risk of complications
- Blood pressure and blood lipids:
  - ◆ Low coronary risk: lifestyle changes only until blood pressure exceeds 160/100. Then use drug therapy with a target of 140/80. Prescribe a statin if cholesterol > 5 mmol/l
  - ◆ High coronary risk: drug therapy when blood pressure exceeds 140/80 mmHg, aiming at 135/75 mmHg. Prescribe a statin if cholesterol > 3 mmol/l. Consider a fibrate if triglycerides > 10 mmol/l

- Recommends full lipid profile on fasting sample
- (NB: These recommendations were published in 2002, since when there has been a trend towards more aggressive treatment)

■ Foot problems:
- Stresses the need for a multidisciplinary team and proposes all patients have their foot risk evaluated
- There are four categories and clear suggestions for the management of patients in each group (for example, see Diabetes Guidelines: Feet, Appendix 2, page 105)

4 Screening and identification

PREVALENCE AND SCREENING

- The prevalence of diabetes in the UK is 3%

- It increases with age: over 7.7% of people aged > 65 have diabetes

- Prevalence in African, Asian and Afro-Caribbean people is > 6%

- Up to 25% of people of Asian origin aged > 60 have diabetes

The most recent Position Statement (2006) from Diabetes UK (available in full on their website) recommends the following people be screened for diabetes:

- White people aged over 40 years and people from Black, Asian and minority ethnic groups aged over 25 with one or more of the risk factors below:

  - A first degree family history of diabetes

  - A BMI of 25–30 kg/m^2 and above, together with a sedentary lifestyle

  - A waist measurement of over 94 cm (37 in) for White and Black men and 80 cm (31.5 in) for White, Black and Asian women, and > 90 cm (35 in) for Asian men

- People who have ischaemic heart disease, cerebrovascular disease, peripheral vascular disease or treated hypertension

- Women who have had gestational diabetes who have tested normal following delivery (screen within 6 weeks of delivery, 1 year post-partum and then 3-yearly)

- Women with polycystic ovary syndrome who have a BMI > 30

- People who are known to have impaired glucose tolerance or impaired fasting glycaemia

- People who have severe mental health problems

- People who have hypertriglyceridemia not due to alcohol excess or renal disease

Other authorities also recommend testing men with erectile dysfunction as this can be the first presenting symptom for type 2 diabetes.

VITAL POINTS

* *People of Asian origin are more likely than others to develop type 2 diabetes, and at an earlier age*
* *Flag the notes of those with a family history of diabetes*
* *Flag the notes of those with a history of gestational diabetes*
* *Screen those at risk of developing diabetes every 3 years*

IDENTIFICATION

- You should 'think diabetes'!
- A practice with 2,000 patients is likely to have 60 people with diabetes
- About 80% of people with diabetes are managed in primary care, ie of 60 patients on your diabetes list, 48 will be managed in your practice
- Of those presenting to your practice with diabetes, many will have diabetes treated with diet and exercise alone. Others will be treated with diet, exercise and a combination of tablets with and without insulin
- Teach administrative staff (clerks/receptionists) about diabetes: to recognise the names of test strips, drugs and insulin on prescriptions, and identify people with diabetes on their notes
- Give responsibility for people with diabetes to a 'named' person in the practice
- Ensure that all staff have appropriate knowledge of diabetes
- Check existing registers
- Check prescription lists
- Check existing 'labelled diabetes' patient records
- Check patients who are new to the practice
- Add newly diagnosed patients to the register

- Be extra vigilant with those treated by diet alone
- Identify the housebound with diabetes – check records
- Display posters in the practice
- Communicate with all members of the primary care team, especially those caring for people who are elderly or have a mental illness or learning difficulty
- Contact the local pharmacist(s); they may know about the local diabetes population

What do you need to know?

- The total population covered by the practice
- The percentage of people aged 65 years or over in the practice
- The ethnic composition of the practice

Finally:

- Add newly identified people with diabetes to your list
- Label the patient records 'Diabetes'
- Use this list as the basis of a diabetes register

WHERE AND HOW PEOPLE PRESENT IN PRIMARY CARE

- At the surgery
- In health promotion clinics
- As new patients to the practice
- At 'home' in screening programmes, eg for older people (> 75)
- At routine medical checks, eg for insurance purposes
- To the community pharmacist, eg presenting with symptoms
- After a visit to the optometrist (optician) for a routine vision check
- At NHS walk-in centres, or via NHS Direct (telephone helpline)
- Self-diagnosis – anywhere

Symptoms of type 2 diabetes: what to look for?

Symptoms (may develop slowly over months or years). They may include some or all of the following:

- Thirst
- Polyuria/nocturia
- Incontinence in elderly people
- Tiredness/lethargy
- Mood changes (irritability)
- Weight loss
- Blurred vision
- Thrush infections (genital)
- Recurrent infections (boils/ulcers)
- Tingling/pain/numbness (in feet, legs, hands)
- Unexplained symptoms

You might want to produce a poster or photocopy the one on page 30 to encourage people with undiagnosed diabetes to come forward. Alternatively, you can obtain such a poster from Diabetes UK (see page 115).

DIAGNOSTIC CRITERIA

Diagnosis of diabetes has important legal and medical implications so diagnosis must be definite:

- Do not base diagnosis on glycosuria or a stick reading of finger-prick blood glucose; use these only for screening
- Measurement of HbAlc is not currently recommended for screening
- Diabetes should be confirmed on a venous plasma blood sample sent to a laboratory. It will be confirmed by:
  - ◆ Random plasma blood glucose concentration of ≥ 11.1 mmol/l, or
  - ◆ Fasting plasma glucose concentration of ≥ 7.0 mmol/l
- Some people with glycosuria have impaired glucose tolerance. This is diagnosed by an OGTT, organised with the local laboratory or in your health centre:

- ♦ Fasting blood glucose, then 75 g glucose or 440 ml of Lucozade
- ♦ Take blood 2 hours later
- ♦ Diabetes = fasting blood glucose ≥ 7.0 and at 2 hours ≥ 11.1 mmol/l
- ♦ Because these results are so important, send blood to the laboratory for glucose measurement, rather than using a glucose meter

■ HbA1c should be measured as a baseline recording

■ Refer children with suspected diabetes urgently: DON'T WAIT for results of diagnostic tests

VITAL POINT

*** If you suspect diabetes in a child, refer them urgently
by telephone to a hospital paediatric department
for confirmation of the diagnosis**

IMPAIRED FASTING GLUCOSE
AND IMPAIRED GLUCOSE TOLERANCE

■ Close monitoring of people with impaired glucose homeostasis is recommended (by the WHO Expert Committee)

■ There are two categories of glucose homeostasis: impaired glucose tolerance (IGT) and a new category of impaired fasting glycaemia (IFG)

■ IGT is defined by a 2-hour glucose during an oral glucose tolerance test (OGTT) of 7.8–11.0 mmol/l, and a fasting plasma glucose of < 7.0 mmol/l

■ IFG is defined by a fasting glucose of 6.1–6.9 mmol/l

■ Two abnormal test results on two different days are needed to confirm the diagnosis. This is important in a patient with no symptoms

■ Those diagnosed as having IGT and IFG are at risk of developing diabetes later in life; they should be advised about lifestyle and dietary points to lessen this risk

■ Such people need to be screened for diabetes every year

■ Screen the same people for cardiovascular disease

DIABETES

DO YOU SUFFER FROM

- Excessive thirst?
- Going to the toilet to pass water (a lot)?
- Blurred vision?
- Itching 'down below'?
- Tiredness?
- Weight loss?
- Mood changes?
- Weight gain?

IF YOU DO, PLEASE LET US KNOW

CRITERIA FOR REFERRAL

Criteria for referral to a diabetes specialist team need to be locally agreed between primary and secondary care providers.

Immediate referral

A person should be referred immediately if:

- They are ill with uncontrolled blood glucose
- They are vomiting continuously
- Tests indicate moderate or heavy ketonuria, or evidence of ketoacidosis
- They have an acutely infected or ischaemic foot
- They are a child with newly diagnosed diabetes

Urgent (within 2 days)

Urgent referral is necessary for people who have:

- Newly diagnosed (type 1) diabetes
- Deteriorating foot problems
- Unexplained loss of vision
- Any woman who is pregnant unexpectedly

Soon (within 1 week)

- Planned pregnancy
- A foot ulcer failing to heal

Routine

Routine referral is necessary for people who have:

- Uncontrolled hypertension

- Sexual dysfunction
- Persistent proteinuria – Albustix positive
- Rising creatinine levels above 120 mmol/l
- Deteriorating retinopathy
- Painful neuropathy, mononeuropathy, amyotrophy
- Psychological problems, such as:
  - Failure to accept diagnosis
  - Morbid fear of complications
  - Family difficulties

VITAL POINT

✱ *Criteria for referral need to be explicitly agreed locally, between primary and secondary care*

BREAKING THE NEWS

- People who have just been told they have a serious illness need time to digest the information
- Explain that diabetes is a life-long condition, and invite them to respond to this
- Find out what they already know about diabetes
- Discuss informally their fears, myths and misconceptions about the condition (see page 43)
- Ask if they know whether anyone in their family suffered from diabetes, and if so, what do they know about how it affected them
- The family, partner or carer needs to be involved in the discussions. So, if the appropriate people are not present, suggest that an early appointment is made for them to attend, especially if they are involved with cooking meals
- Remember that the person's perception of diabetes will affect how they cope in this period immediately after diagnosis

- Explain the symptoms of diabetes and assure them that these can be quickly relieved; diabetes is a controllable long-term condition

- Provide non-judgmental and positive ongoing support to people with diabetes and their families

- Give a simple explanation of the physiology of diabetes and its treatment at an early appointment

- Discuss home monitoring of urine and blood glucose (see Appendix 1)

- Reinforce patients' desire to take care of themselves

- Arrange the next appointment

VITAL POINTS

* *Don't bombard a patient with information*
* *Give plenty of time for him or her to deal with it*

The text that follows (and all pages headed 'Patient and carer information') can be copied and given to patients so that they know what to expect, and what is expected of them

- If you have type 2 diabetes, you will have too much sugar (glucose) in your blood because your body is unable to use it properly

- Insulin is the hormone that helps the glucose to make its way into the cells where it can be used for energy

- Insulin also stops your liver from producing too much glucose

- The main symptoms are being very thirsty, needing to pass urine often, feeling extremely tired, weight loss, general itching and blurred vision

- Type 2 diabetes develops either when your body does not produce enough insulin, or when the insulin produced does not work properly (insulin resistance)

- The main aims of treatment are:
  - To achieve near normal blood sugar (glucose) levels by living a healthy lifestyle which will help you to feel better
  - To improve your blood pressure by ensuring that it is checked and that you are taking any prescribed tablets
  - To protect you against long-term damage to the eyes, kidneys, nerves, heart and major arteries (blood vessels)

- Once you have been diagnosed as having type 2 diabetes, you should have:
  - A full medical examination
  - A talk with a registered nurse with a special interest in diabetes
  - A talk with a state-registered dietitian
  - A discussion about the implications of your diabetes for your job, driving, insurance and prescription charges
  - Information about Diabetes UK, their services and your local group
  - Continuing education about your diabetes

- Depending on your treatment, you should also have the following:
  - If you are treated with diet alone, instructions on blood or urine tests and how to interpret the results, and supplies of equipment

- If you are treated with tablets, the above plus additional discussions about hypoglycaemia ('hypos' = low blood sugar) and how to deal with them
- If you are treated with insulin, both of the above plus a session on injection technique, looking after insulin and injection devices, and also blood sugar (glucose) testing
- Information about what can happen to your diabetes control if you become ill

THE METABOLIC SYNDROME

Also known as Reaven's syndrome or insulin resistance syndrome, this is a complex condition associated with:

- Insulin resistance and type 2 diabetes
- Hypertension
- Central obesity
- Hyperlipidaemia (low HDL cholesterol : high LDL cholesterol)
- Hyperinsulinaemia
- Polycystic ovary syndrome

At the heart of this syndrome is the problem of insulin resistance. This is a vicious circle: insulin resistance can lead to weight gain, which in turn worsens insulin resistance.

Insulin resistance

- Insulin resistance is one of the fundamental defects of type 2 diabetes
- Insulin resistance is an early feature of the development of type 2 diabetes
- The body fails to respond to its own insulin. Initially, this can be compensated for by an increase in insulin secretion
- Insulin-resistant patients may become hyperinsulinaemic
- Continued insulin resistance leads eventually to exhaustion of the pancreatic beta cells. This results in a failure to produce adequate insulin and a further increase in blood glucose
- In type 2 diabetes, insulin resistance is characterised by:
  - ◆ Impaired (insulin-stimulated) glucose uptake by fat, liver and skeletal muscle
  - ◆ Over-production of glucose by the liver

- Insulin resistance is central to the development of cardiovascular risk factors, which are clustered together in the metabolic syndrome described earlier

- Regular vigorous exercise improves oxygen consumption and reduces insulin resistance – even in elderly people

- Problems caused by insulin resistance can be reduced by lifestyle changes

- Thiazolidinediones (also called PPAR-gamma agonists, glitazones or insulin sensitisers) are drugs that target insulin resistance. They improve glycaemic control by improving insulin sensitivity at key sites of insulin resistance – namely fat, liver and skeletal muscle

- Thiazolidinediones are not licensed for the treatment of impaired glucose tolerance (IGT) or impaired fasting glycaemia (IFG). However, a recent study with rosiglitazone (Gerstain *et al* 2006) showed a 60% reduction in the development of diabetes in this group

VITAL POINT

* *Insulin resistance is one of the fundamental defects of type 2 diabetes*

HYPERTENSION

- Raised blood pressure is very common in type 2 diabetes (up to 50%)

- There is increasing evidence that aggressive BP treatment reduces vascular complications in diabetes

- As a result, the threshold for starting treatment and the target for treatment are both falling

- Start treatment if systolic BP > 150 or diastolic BP > 90 mmHg

- Aim at normalising blood pressure (130/80)

- Treat older people with equal enthusiasm, because they are more likely to derive early benefit

Drugs used to treat hypertension

- There is evidence that ACE (angiotensin-converting enzyme) inhibitors have a protective effect on kidneys in people with diabetes, and possibly reduce retinopathy over and above their effect in reducing blood pressure

- There is additional evidence that ARBs (angiotensin receptor blockers, sartans) are particularly good at protecting the kidney in diabetes

- The UKPDS (UK Prospective Diabetes Study, see page 12) found that ACE inhibitors confer no greater benefit than beta blockers in hypertension. However, the UKPDS carries the simple messages:
  - High BP is common in type 2 diabetes
  - Tight BP control has a major effect in reducing complications, including retinopathy
  - Many patients need two or more drugs to achieve the target BP of 130/80

- Doctors should use the antihypertensive drugs they are familiar with, remembering that (in hypertension) concordance with treatment may be improved if a drug needs to be taken only once a day

- All drugs used for treating hypertension have well-recognised side effects:
  - Thiazides – low serum K^+, raised blood glucose and impotence
  - Beta blockers – may worsen asthma
  - ACE inhibitors – cough; and in rare cases they can cause renal failure or angioneurotic oedema
  - Calcium blockers – flushing, headache, oedema

Risk factors for coronary heart disease

- The major risk factors for CHD are:
  - Increased LDL cholesterol concentration
  - Decreased HDL cholesterol concentration
  - Hyperglycaemia (HbA1c > 6.2%)
  - Insulin resistance
  - Hypertension
  - Smoking
  - Being male

* *Educate patients about the importance of BP in diabetes*
* *Check BP at every clinic visit in all patients – especially if there is proteinuria*
* *Aim for a target BP of 130/80 mmHg*

ASSESSING AND EXAMINING

THE NEWLY DIAGNOSED PATIENT

Assessment, examination and tests for a newly diagnosed person with diabetes should be sensitive to the individual and carried out in stages.

Stage 1

- Discuss general aspects of diabetes:
  - Ask about any family history
  - Ask about history of illness leading to diagnosis
- Listen and respond to preconceived ideas and anxieties. Establish the person's existing knowledge of diabetes
- Give a simple explanation of diabetes, discuss any fears that the patient may have, and answer questions
- Discuss the patient's general health and make the next appointment

Stage 2

- Discuss all results from the patient's previous visit and lifestyle in relation to diabetes; record drinking and smoking, advise strongly against the latter
- Weigh the patient and measure height. Calculate body mass index (BMI) and agree target for body weight:

    BMI = Weight in kilograms/(Height in metres)^2, that is kg/m^2

- Measure blood pressure
- Examine the patient for complications of diabetes:
  - Lower limbs

- ◆ Peripheral pulses and sensation
- ◆ Visual acuity
- ◆ Fundoscopy with dilated pupils

■ Enrol the patient in a retinal screening programme

■ Test urine for glucose, ketones and protein. Send sample for microalbuminuria

■ Test blood for fasting glucose, renal function, HbA1c

■ Measure fasting cholesterol and triglyceride levels; this should be done after a period of treatment because initial high triglycerides may improve with better blood glucose control

■ Consider arranging the following tests and reconsider at each annual review:
- ◆ Full blood count
- ◆ ECG
- ◆ Liver function tests
- ◆ Thyroid function tests

Stage 3

■ Discuss all results from the patient's previous visit and lifestyle in relation to diabetes; record drinking and smoking, advise strongly against the latter

■ Discuss food and meal planning. Initiate advice about eating plan

■ Arrange prescription (if required) and next appointment – regular and early reviews will be necessary until the patient has a good understanding of diabetes and metabolic control is achieved

■ Record information in the practice records and in diabetes cooperation cards, if used

■ Enter patient details on practice diabetes register, and notify information to district diabetes register. (Patients must be informed if data are held on a register outside the practice)

Assessment checklist at diagnosis and annual review

The following information should be checked and recorded:

■ Demographic information

    ◆ Any changes?   *Yes* ☐   *No* ☐

■ Family status

    ◆ Any changes?   *Yes* ☐   *No* ☐

■ Employment status

    ◆ Any changes?   *Yes* ☐   *No* ☐

■ Medical history

    ◆ Any changes?   *Yes* ☐   *No* ☐

■ Lifestyle history

    ◆ Any changes?   *Yes* ☐   *No* ☐

■ Diabetes management

    ◆ Any changes?   *Yes* ☐   *No* ☐

VITAL POINTS

✽ Time spent educating the patient is an investment in preventing complications and maintaining well-being in the future

✽ A trusting, therapeutic relationship is vital to encourage continuity of health care

- Find out all you can about diabetes and check the information with your care team
- Tell other people about your diabetes: your family, friends and work colleagues
- Attend for regular checks
- Be in control of your diabetes on a daily basis
- Monitor your own sugar levels and change treatment as advised
- Keep a record of your blood (or urine) tests
- Know when to seek help and where, particularly in an emergency or if you are ill
- Discuss your fears with your team
- Ask questions and repeat them if you don't get an answer. Prepare them before your appointment
- Follow a healthy lifestyle:
  - Choose healthy food
  - Keep your weight at a sensible level
  - Take regular physical exercise
  - Don't smoke!
- Examine your feet regularly. If you find this difficult, try to arrange for someone else to do this
- Recognise signs of low/high blood glucose levels, and make sure you know how to prevent them getting out of control
- Be aware of the long-term complications of diabetes, the importance of early detection and the relevance of reducing blood glucose (sugar) levels to reduce the risk of complications
- Inform the DVLA (tel: 0870 240 0009) and your insurance company if you drive
- Carry personal identification (Medic-Alert) and warning card with details of who can help
- If you are female and hoping to have a baby, get advice on your diabetes before trying to conceive
- Consider joining Diabetes UK to keep you updated about diabetes

- Management in primary care should include the following actions:
  - Give a full medical examination on diagnosis
  - Give all patients with diabetes an annual review, including the measurement of HbA1c and screening for complications
  - Review all patients with diabetes every 3–6 months to assess control of blood glucose, blood pressure and side effects of treatment
- Management aims should include:
  - Relief of symptoms
  - Discussion of potential side effects of treatment, especially hypos
  - Reduction in risks of acute complications
  - Identification of long-term complications (as early as possible)
  - Ensuring the patient has a satisfactory lifestyle
- Offer support, advice and education about treatment to all patients with diabetes
- Negotiate appropriate targets for control and treatment
- Assess the symptoms and well-being of individuals with diabetes on a regular basis
- Provide initial and continuing education to people with diabetes and their carers
- Provide information about social and economic support

Routine review

- Ensure that patients with established diabetes are included on the diabetes register and are booked for regular appointments
- Organise a system for identifying and recalling defaulters, and agree a policy for the frequency of follow-up of people with diabetes
- Routine visits may be required 2–3 times a year in patients whose management and understanding of the condition are established
- Make time to discuss the patient's attitude to diabetes and general well-being; ask about any problems (life changes, hypos, diet, etc)
- If the patient is treated with insulin, check injection sites

- Most patients will have times in their life when their diabetes is difficult to control, ie family crises, other health problems, etc. Identify those who may be having problems on a regular basis and discuss with the patient how to deal with this

- Check the patient's weight and blood pressure. Start treatment if blood pressure is raised

- Test urine for glucose, ketones and albumin; check mid-stream urine (MSU) if albumin is present

- Take a blood sample for HbA1c. It makes sense to take this, and any other blood samples, 7 days before review appointments so that results are available in time for discussion with the patient

- Identify and discuss any weak spots in the patient's knowledge of diabetes and self management skills

- Make it clear that the patient should return if there are problems with hypos, high sugar levels or side effects. Set agreed limits to blood glucose levels

- Discuss and agree targets with the patient relating to their records of blood or urine tests, altering therapy as required

- Record all details in diabetes record card and/or practice record

- Arrange the next appointment

VITAL POINT

* Patients who take part in regular structured care have better metabolic control and less risk of complications

Annual review

- Refer to local guidelines if they are in place (see Appendix 2)

- Enquire about life events and ask if the patient has experienced any of the following:
  - ◆ Subjective changes in eyes and feet
  - ◆ Claudication
  - ◆ Neuropathic symptoms, including impotence
  - ◆ Chest pain, shortness of breath

- Weigh the patient and discuss general progress and well-being; enquire about any problems relating to diabetes, in particular hypos or side effects of drugs

- If the patient is treated with insulin, check injection sites

- Test urine for glucose, albumin and ketones. Check for micro-albuminuria

- Arrange MSU if albumin or blood is present

- Examine for diabetic complications:
  - Blood pressure
  - Visual acuity
  - Eyes: refer for screening
  - Arrange MSU, if appropriate
  - Feet: general condition, pulses, ulceration, sensation

- Review and agree targets with the patient relating to their blood (or urine) tests

- Take blood sample for the following tests, which should be performed in advance of the annual review:
  - Blood glucose (feed back result)
  - HbA1c
  - Creatinine (see Appendix 3)
  - Cholesterol (see Appendix 3)

- Check and discuss management with the patient under the following headings:
  - Dietary concerns
  - Treatment
  - Targets
  - Risk factors for heart disease and other long-term complications
  - Management plan, including contraception and plans for pregnancies in women – altering therapy as required

- Record information in the records, practice diabetes register and patient cooperation card if used

- Arrange prescription (if required) and next appointment

- Notify information to the District Diabetes Register

Once your diabetes is controlled:

■ You should be able to see the diabetes team regularly and be able to discuss problems and diabetes control

■ You should also be able to get in touch with any member of the team for specialist advice

■ You will have more education sessions

■ You will attend a medical review with a doctor or trained nurse once a year; this will involve the following:

- ◆ Being weighed

- ◆ A urine test for protein and microalbuminuria

- ◆ A blood test to check long-term glucose control

- ◆ A blood pressure measurement

- ◆ Blood tests for HbA1c (glucose control), cholesterol and creatinine

- ◆ Discussion about glucose control

- ◆ Discussion about treatment for blood pressure and cholesterol

- ◆ A vision check and photograph of the back of your eyes; if significant problems are found you will be referred to an ophthalmologist (eye specialist)

- ◆ Examination of your feet

- ◆ Discussion of the impact of diabetes at home and at work

6 Educating patients about managing type 2 diabetes

It is important to recognise that, in all long-term disease, myths and misconceptions, preconceived ideas, education and life experience form the basis of individual health beliefs. This is particularly true at the time of diagnosis, when attitudes to the concept of a life-long incurable medical condition are set into place.

In diabetes, myths and misconceptions abound. Acknowledging and dispelling them is the first step in educating patients.

MYTHS AND MISCONCEPTIONS

- Diabetes can be cured
- Type 2 diabetes is a 'mild' condition
- It is caused by eating too much sugar
- It is the patient's fault
- Dietary treatment means severe restriction
- Specialist diabetic foods will be essential
- If insulin is required, the diabetes is more severe

ENCOURAGING SELF-MANAGEMENT

- Self-management education is considered to be a fundamental part of diabetes care
- NICE and the NSF have recommended that structured patient education is made available from diagnosis to all people with diabetes

DESMOND (Diabetes Education and Self-Management Ongoing and Newly Diagnosed)

- The DESMOND initiative brings together a multidisciplinary team of health care professionals and people with diabetes from different health care settings across England

- The group has developed a new curriculum for people recently diagnosed with type 2 diabetes

- This is based on principles of adult learning and is being tested by a randomised controlled trial

- The aim of the group is to develop DESMOND modules for ongoing care and to train educators in each health community

EDUCATION CHECKLIST:

THE PRIMARY CARE TEAM

The following topics should be discussed with patients:

- What is diabetes?
- Diet
- Tablets
- Insulin and injection technique
- Hypoglycaemia
- Hyperglycaemia
- Illness
- Blood testing
- Urine testing
- Foot care
- Importance of eye checks
- Smoking
- Alcohol
- Exercise
- Complications
- Driving and insurance

- Sexual health
- Planning pregnancy
- Diabetes UK
- Free prescriptions
- Benefits

Although most patients can control their blood glucose by diet and/or tablets at the onset, this becomes more difficult with time. This is a result of beta-cell failure and progressive insulin resistance and is not the patient's fault. Most people with type 2 diabetes end up needing insulin; the average time from diagnosis is 6 years.

VITAL POINTS

* *Teaching patients how to manage their own diabetes is an essential part of care*
* *Patients should be warned that they are likely to need insulin therapy in time, and that this is in no way their fault*

CULTURAL ISSUES

- Be aware of different cultures and religions and the effect these have on diabetes care, such as your approach to a patient on initial presentation and advice about diet and lifestyle
- Be aware of the differences in etiquette when examining patients from different cultures
- Respect the individual's culture and lifestyle
- Find out how to communicate with patients from ethnic minorities as well as about their customs and dietary rules
- There are many cultural differences with regard to food and these need to be remembered when the person with diabetes is from a different culture
- Be aware that in some communities it is believed that certain foods are 'hot' whereas others are 'cold' – during certain illnesses, only one type will be eaten

- Remember that people from some ethnic minorities have particular dietary habits and eat foods that are of cultural importance, eg ghee and sweetmeats among Asian communities (Hindu and Muslim), halal meat (Muslim), kosher food (Jewish), etc. These need to be incorporated into dietary advice
- There is evidence that fasting (eg during Ramadan) leads to erratic blood glucose levels. Discuss the details of fasting with your patient and try to devise a treatment plan which covers eating after sundown. PPGRs (page 59) may help
- Some traditional/herbal medicines used in certain Afro-Asian communities may cause hypoglycaemia or liver damage. Ask patients about their use
- Try to organise a link worker for different ethnic groups
- In some cultures, the idea of self-injection is anathema. Take this into consideration and suggest a third party takes responsibility for insulin injections

VITAL POINT

* Respecting patients' culture and lifestyles is an important step in providing appropriate care. Patients are less likely to concord with treatment they find inappropriate

General advice

■ You have a vital part to play in your own treatment and management:
- ◆ Eat regular meals
- ◆ Avoid being overweight
- ◆ Eat more high-fibre and starchy foods, such as wholemeal bread and cereals
- ◆ Eat less in the way of sugary foods, such as sweetened drinks, cakes and chocolate
- ◆ Cut down on the amount of fat you eat
- ◆ Go easy on the amount of salt you use
- ◆ Drink alcohol in moderation only
- ◆ Avoid special 'diabetic' products – they can be high in fat and cost more
- ◆ DO NOT SMOKE
- ◆ Take regular exercise

■ If you follow the above, by healthy eating and exercise, you will be able to lower your blood sugar (glucose) levels

■ By keeping your blood glucose levels in the normal range you will reduce the risk of complications of diabetes

■ If your blood glucose levels remain above target, you will need insulin – with or without tablets

■ Check your feet and footwear regularly and keep your feet clean

■ Get your eyes checked regularly:
- ◆ You are entitled to a free eye check every year if you take tablets or insulin for your diabetes
- ◆ You should have an annual eye photograph

■ Know what to do if you are ill or have hypoglycaemia (a hypo)
- ◆ You do not have to pay for prescriptions if you are on tablets or insulin

Meal planning advice

This list gives advice about the way in which your meals should be planned:

- Maintain a constant intake of energy (ie eat regularly) as fluctuations have an effect on blood glucose levels

- Eat regular meals

- Cut back on foods that are high in energy, including fatty meat, fried foods, dairy products. Sugary foods and drinks result in poor blood sugar (glucose) control

- Half your energy intake should come from starches such as bread, potatoes, rice, pasta, cereals, beans and lentils

- Eat high-fibre foods (such as whole-grain bread, jacket potatoes)

- Beans, lentils and oats have been shown to promote a slow, steadier rise in blood sugar levels

- Keep carbohydrates such as sweets, chocolates and sweet drinks for special occasions, emergencies such as hypoglycaemia (hypo) or illness, or as a snack before strenuous activity

- Ask your diabetes team for advice if you need to lose weight; work with a dietitian or practice nurse to plan your meals

- Eat less fat and cut down on salt

- Control your alcohol intake: a maximum of three 'units' for men and two for women per day is recommended (1 'unit' = half pint of ordinary beer or lager or small glass of wine or a single measure of spirits)

- Don't buy special diabetic foods:
  - They are expensive and often high in fat
  - They may contain sorbitol, which can cause diarrhoea

Weight control advice

- The more weight you carry, the greater the problem with insulin resistance, which leads to increased glucose levels. Even a small weight reduction can improve this

- By keeping your weight down, you may put off the need for tablets, as diabetes can be controlled by diet for longer
- You can control your weight through diet and through exercise or activity
- Itemise your diet and discuss with the appropriate experts how you can adjust it to help you meet your goals/targets
- Ask for help and encouragement from family and friends
- Find a realistic routine that suits you
- Enjoy what you do eat, and make allowances for occasional lapses
- If you aim to lose weight, you may need to reduce your tablets/insulin. Discuss this with your diabetes care team

Exercise/activity advice

- The Health Education Authority recommends that you have 30 minutes of moderate physical exercise/activity on at least 5 days a week
- This will improve your health
- Build up to this target gradually, over 3 or 4 weeks
- Consider ways of making exercise part of your daily routine
- Moderate activity is activity that raises your heartbeat and makes you feel warm and slightly out of breath (with the emphasis on 'slightly')
- Physical activity includes gardening, brisk walking, cycling, swimming, dancing and various sports
- Do not take up strenuous activity unless you have been examined by a doctor and pronounced fit
- By exercising and improving your health, you can:
  - Manage the stresses of life
  - Control your blood pressure
  - Reduce your risk of heart disease
  - Prevent brittle bones in later life
  - Reduce the risks of some cancers
  - Keep mobile and independent in later life

Alcohol advice

■ Alcohol reduces the production of glucose by the liver for up to 12 hours, even though the level of sugar in the bloodstream may rise immediately after drinking alcohol with high carbohydrate levels

■ All the rules about alcohol that apply to everyone apply to you

■ Too much alcohol (whether high carbohydrate ones such as beer and lager or those containing no carbohydrates such as spirits or low-calorie mixers) may cause a hypo, particularly if you take insulin

■ Alcohol always contains calories so heavy drinking will make you overweight, leading to poor sugar (glucose) control and poor health, with the continuing risk of a hypo

■ If and when you drink, avoid low-sugar beers which are higher in alcohol content and low-alcohol beers which are high in sugar; go for ordinary beers, and avoid drinks that are high in sugar (sweet wine/sherry/liqueurs)

■ Use mixers or soft drinks that are diet, low calorie or sugar free

■ Know your drinks and check the percentage alcohol content

■ Limit your drinking to two (women) or three (men) units a day (1 unit = half a pint of beer, a glass of wine or a single pub measure of spirits)

■ If you take insulin, don't drink on an empty stomach

■ Eat little and often while you are drinking

■ Always carry glucose tablets or sweets

■ Always wear or carry your diabetes information as a hypo can be confused with drunkenness

■ Hypos can happen the morning after an evening drinking session

■ Avoid alcohol if you are pregnant as it could harm your baby

7 Longer term management of type 2 diabetes

In the longer term, treatment of diabetes has the following aims:

- Relief of symptoms
- Allowing the person to maintain a satisfactory lifestyle
- Prevention of unwanted effects of treatment (ie hypoglycaemia, side effects of drugs)
- Reduction of the risks of acute complications (hypoglycaemia, hyperglycaemia)
- Reduction of the risks of long-term complications including coronary heart disease, visual impairment, amputation and renal failure

TARGETS FOR GOOD
BLOOD GLUCOSE CONTROL

- The targets for good diabetic control are fasting blood glucose (FBG, finger prick test) < 6 mmol/l and HbA1c < 7%
- The UKPDS has demonstrated two important points:
  - Patients who achieve these targets have a lower risk of developing complications
  - Type 2 diabetes is a progressive disorder caused by insulin resistance and increasing loss of insulin production by the pancreas
- Total blood glucose load over time is a major risk factor for vascular disease and diabetic complications
- At the onset, patients find it easy to control blood glucose within tight limits
- UKPDS has shown that most patients progress from a single tablet regimen, through to combination regimens and inevitably to insulin therapy to ensure tight glycaemic control

- The average time from diagnosis to needing insulin is 6 years. Goals are set for patients, which are increasingly hard to achieve because of risk or fear of hypos or unacceptable weight gain

- Patients need to be told this sobering information and reassured that, when and if they come to need insulin, it is because their diabetes is getting worse and not through any fault of their own

VITAL POINTS

* **Type 2 diabetes is a progressive condition**
* **Diet is the first line treatment for type 2 diabetes**
* **Avoid tablets for the first 3 months, unless the patient is very symptomatic or blood glucose exceeds 15 mmol/l**

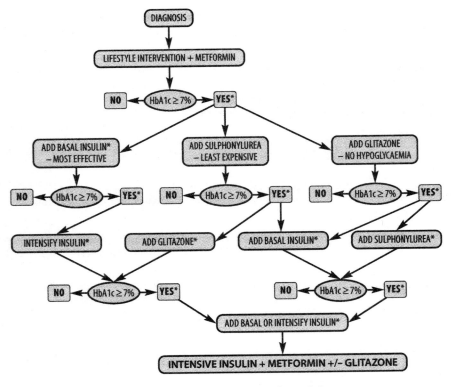

ADA EASD Guideline, reproduced with permission

TREATMENT PLAN FOR TYPE 2 DIABETES

■ Given the progressive nature of type 2 diabetes, patients tend to feel that they have let us – or themselves – down when they are unable to maintain tight blood glucose control

TREATMENT WITH TABLETS

Metformin

■ First-line treatment especially in **overweight patients** with type 2 diabetes

■ Shown in UKPDS to have positive effects on cardiovascular outcomes

■ Main action is to decrease hepatic glucose output

■ Side effects are common and occur in 30% of patients prescribed metformin, and include nausea, flatulence, diarrhoea, constipation, anorexia, metallic taste and impaired absorption of vitamin B12

■ Take with food to minimise side effects

■ Start with one tablet a day and increase the dose at weekly intervals

■ Lactic acidosis is a very rare but serious complication

■ Avoid in cardiac failure or renal impairment (creatinine > 130 μmol/l)

■ Avoid in women who are pregnant or breast-feeding

VITAL POINT

* Avoid metformin in people with failure of the heart, kidneys or liver

Sulphonylureas

■ Often used in **normal weight patients** with type 2 diabetes

■ Stimulate insulin release from the pancreas

■ Potent drugs, which may cause profound hypoglycaemia, particularly when first introduced

■ If hypoglycaemia occurs, reduce the dose

- May induce weight gain, as a result of the anabolic effect of insulin

- Avoid in women who are pregnant or breast-feeding

- Use with caution in elderly people with diabetes and those with renal failure

- Side effects are mild and infrequent: rashes, headache and, very rarely, blood disorders

- Glibenclamide is not often used because of the risk of dangerous long-lasting hypos

- Gliclazide is safer in renal failure and appears to cause fewer hypos in elderly people with diabetes

- Glimepiride is a new generation, long-acting, single-dose sulphonylurea. It has the advantage of being taken as a single dose

VITAL POINTS

* *Avoid all tablets in pregnant women*
* *All sulphonylureas can cause hypos*

Insulin sensitisers (thiazolidinediones)

- Licensed as:
  - Monotherapy (particularly in the overweight); patients for whom metformin is inappropriate due to contraindications or intolerance
  - Dual therapy with metformin for those with insufficient control on maximum tolerated dose of metformin
  - Dual therapy with a sulphonylurea, if patient intolerant to or contraindicated for metformin if insufficient control is seen
  - Triple therapy with metformin and a sulphonylurea, if control is insufficient

- Act by improving insulin resistance, the root cause of type 2 diabetes

- Reduce blood glucose and insulin levels by increasing effectiveness of available insulin in liver, fat and muscle

- Potentiate the action of both the body's own insulin and also injected insulin

- Rosiglitazone was launched in the UK in July 2000. Initial liver function testing is recommended, as is periodic testing thereafter. It can be used in combination with metformin or sulphonylureas, but is contraindicated for use in combination with insulin

- Pioglitazone was launched in November 2000. Use is as for rosiglitazone. The Proactive study of pioglitazone to reduce CV risk factors failed to show a reduction in its primary endpoint. However, there was a significant reduction in the combined endpoint of MI or cardiovascular death

- Thiazolidinediones are well tolerated and, because of their mechanism of action, have a low risk of hypos when given as monotherapy

- Evidence has accumulated that glitazones have added positive benefits on blood pressure and a range of cardiovascular risk factors

- Side effects are minimal in patients without cardiovascular problems. Side effects include weight gain and ankle swelling (dilutional anaemia) unrelated to heart failure

- In patients with heart failure, fluid retention associated with glitazones may cause decompensation. Thus, glitazones should be avoided

VITAL POINT

✶ Glitazones should be avoided in all patients with known heart failure

Postprandial glucose regulators

- Postprandial glucose regulators (PPGRs, eg repaglinide) are taken immediately before a meal

- If a meal is missed, then it is not necessary to take a dose

- PPGRs work like a sulphonylurea, with a faster onset and shorter duration of action

- They can be introduced when diet and exercise are no longer adequate

- They can be used when metformin monotherapy is insufficient

- Incidence of hypos is less with PPGRs than with sulphonylureas

Combination of drugs

- Since type 2 diabetes is a progressive disease, combination therapy is seen as the preferred method of treatment for maintaining good glycaemic control

- Combination therapy with metformin and a glitazone may be particularly appropriate in the overweight

- Triple combination therapy with metformin, sulphonylurea, glitazone has become an accepted part of clinical practice and provides an interim alternative to insulin

- A combination of metformin and a thiazolidinedione or a sulphonylurea and a thiazolidinedione is approved by NICE

- Metformin causes gastrointestinal side effects (wind, nausea and – rarely – constipation). People often feel better after starting insulin

- The UKPDS demonstrated the importance of tight blood glucose control in reducing or delaying long-term complications of type 2 diabetes. Thus patients with HbA1c > 7.5% on a combination of tablets should consider the need for insulin

- People with diabetes often have other risk factors, such as hypertension or raised lipids, and need to take additional medication to reduce these risks

- Tablet boxes to organise daily medication are available from chemists

VITAL POINTS

* *The UKPDS showed that tight blood glucose control is important in reducing or delaying long-term complications of type 2 diabetes*

* *It does not matter how this is achieved*

* *Any reduction in glycated haemoglobin (HbA1c) will be beneficial in the reduction of long-term complications*

* *Don't be afraid to try any combination of therapies to achieve the desired result*

Combination with insulin

- Traditionally, people with type 2 diabetes have been treated with tablets for as long as possible, and then changed over to insulin

- A new and acceptable approach is combination therapy with tablets and insulin

- This helps people become accustomed to insulin injections and to adjusting the dose according to their blood glucose tests

- Start by adding a long-acting insulin at bedtime (say 10 units) and monitoring the early morning glucose

- The final dose of insulin needed to achieve a morning glucose < 6 mmol/l will depend mainly on body weight

- The dose of insulin should be increased steadily until the target is achieved

- Metformin or sulphonylureas should be continued at the previous dose, which should be more effective if the fasting glucose is well controlled

- As the beta cells in the pancreas cease to function, daytime blood glucose levels will creep up, resulting in a rise in HbA1c

- At some stage, tablets have little useful effect and the person will have to move over to two or more daily injections of insulin

Note that, at each stage in this process, the person with diabetes and the clinic team must decide whether or not to move on to the next stage:

- Many people, particularly if they are elderly or very overweight, may be better off accepting less than ideal metabolic control

- In the UKPDS, the benefits of tight control were not seen for about 6 years

- So, in people with a life expectancy shorter than this, there is no point in struggling for perfection

VITAL POINT

✱ Combination therapy with a bedtime dose of insulin suits many people – it provides a gentle introduction to full-blown insulin therapy

- Insulin therapy should be considered in type 2 diabetes when:
  - Symptoms persist
  - Blood glucose levels are high – HbA1c > 7.5%
  - There is an intercurrent illness or a need for steroid therapy
- Decision to move over to insulin therapy:
- When there are symptoms of thirst, tiredness, itchy genitalia
- Depends on body weight: it is difficult to treat very obese patients with insulin
- Predictors of successful insulin therapy:
  - When a person is committed to good control
  - Depends on family history: parents or siblings are on insulin
  - When workmates or friends are on insulin – they may encourage someone to 'take the plunge'
- HbA1c is the best indicator of metabolic control. Inform patients of the local threshold and about progressive loss of insulin production by the pancreas
- Treatment with insulin should start with a small dose of insulin – usually 10 units twice daily of long-acting or pre-mixed insulin
- Overweight patients will need larger doses
- Those who measure their own blood glucose can be taught to increase their dose in response to the level. They may want to discuss changes with their care team
- Most people with type 2 diabetes achieve satisfactory control with twice daily insulin; a few need three or four daily injections

Practical details regarding the use and adjustment of insulin are not given here because of space limitations, but there is a great deal of information available in the book by Rosemary Walker and Jill Rodgers (see page 113).

VITAL POINT

* The decision to change to insulin is a process that may take several months

UNDERSTANDING HYPERGLYCAEMIA

- Hyperglycaemia is arbitarily defined as a glucose level of > 12 mmol/l

- It can result from non-concordance with treatment

- Most patients forget to take their tablets/insulin from time to time. If one dose of tablets/insulin is forgotten within 1 hour of the usual time, take as usual. If longer than this, omit the dose and take the usual dose when the next one is due. DO NOT double the following dose. Accept that blood glucose levels will be temporarily raised

- Hyperglycaemia may be caused by:
  - Untreated diabetes
  - Too much food
  - The wrong type of food
  - Infections or other illness
  - Insufficient tablets or insulin (incorrect dose)
  - Overuse of particular injection sites – leading to fatty lumps
  - Poor injection technique
  - Reduction of activity
  - An increase in drugs affecting glycaemic control (eg steroid therapy)
  - Stress leading to lifestyle changes
  - Weight increase

Monitoring hyperglycaemia

- People with diabetes should become accustomed to monitoring their own health, provided they are capable. You will need to support and go through their self-monitoring records with them

- Patients should monitor their own general health, well-being, diabetes control, eyesight, weight, dental care, care of the feet and footwear

- To promote health and reduce risks of complications, you should teach them how to monitor their diabetes control by testing their blood glucose

- Monitoring allows them to check their own control, take responsibility for their condition and, as far as possible, maintain independence

- If you suspect that the person with diabetes has hypoglycaemia (from discussion of symptoms or reports of 'dizzy spells'), blood glucose levels should be checked and medication or insulin reduced

- Hyperglycaemic episodes will require an increase in tablets or insulin

- You will have to decide with the patient whether any change in therapy is needed, eg diet alone to tablet therapy to combination tablet therapy to combination tablet plus insulin therapy to insulin therapy – all in association with dietary guidelines

- Decisions about adding tablets or insulin should be taken in consultation with the person with diabetes

- By monitoring dietary habits, changes in weight, lifestyle and other medical problems (particularly in elderly people), you can decide when review of treatment is necessary

VITAL POINTS

* *It is important that people with diabetes are taught how to monitor their own diabetes*

* *Persistent hyperglycaemia points to the need for a change in therapy*

General

■ Occasional high sugar tests (hyperglycaemia) can be ignored

■ However, you should look out for symptoms of hyperglycaemia:
  ◆ Thirst
  ◆ Passing urine frequently, particularly at night
  ◆ Lethargy/tiredness
  ◆ Irritability
  ◆ Blurred vision

■ Persistent hyperglycaemia requires adjustment of food, activity, medication and/or insulin

■ If you are ill or have an infection, your blood sugar (glucose) is likely to climb. If so, contact your GP or care team

■ If you are ill and vomiting, treat this as a medical emergency and summon urgent help

Urine testing

■ Urine testing is important and gives you information about your sugar (glucose) levels

■ If you are unsure of how this is done, then ask at your surgery

■ Urine testing is inexpensive

■ You can get urine testing strips on prescription. You will have to pay for these if you are treated by diet alone

■ Testing and recording your sugar levels helps you control your diabetes

■ Testing a freshly passed urine specimen before breakfast (but not the first one of the day) indicates whether control is good

■ Testing about 2 hours after a meal indicates your highest urinary sugar (glucose) levels

- Aim at negative urine tests first thing in the morning and 0–1% after food
- You need a watch or clock with a second hand for home urine testing
- You should be taught how to record tests and be provided with a testing diary – ask your care team

Blood testing

- Confirmation of improved blood sugar (glucose) levels will encourage you to continue with your self-care, treatment and monitoring
- Blood glucose levels will improve if you can lose weight
- Many people on tablets for their diabetes like to test their blood glucose for information about their own diabetes, particularly if they suspect hypos or have high blood glucose levels
- It is important to keep records of all your results. Only in this way will you be able to detect patterns of blood glucose levels that may require a change in medication

If you have type 2 diabetes and are on tablets or insulin, you are exempt from prescription charges.

UNDERSTANDING HYPOGLYCAEMIA

- Hypoglycaemia means a blood glucose level < 3.5 mmol/l
- Symptoms of hypoglycaemia may be experienced at levels > 3.5 mmol/l, when blood glucose levels have been high over a long period of time (eg immediately after diagnosis). This is temporary and will disappear once blood glucose levels settle
- Hypoglycaemia is more likely to occur in those who have strict control of their blood glucose levels
- Hypoglycaemia is more common soon after starting a sulphonylurea
- In elderly people, hypoglycaemia resulting from sulphonylureas carries a high mortality rate. Symptoms may persist for 24 hours. Once it is diagnosed, consider hospitalisation

- If the patient on a sulphonylurea has problems with hypoglycaemia, consider a change to a thiazolidinedione or postprandial glucose regulator (PPGR)

Monitoring hypoglycaemia

- Hypoglycaemia may occur several hours after extra activity
- Hypoglycaemia may be caused by:
  - Too little food (especially in elderly people)
  - Delayed or missed meals
  - Increased medication or insulin
  - Increased activity (exercise)
  - Increased mobility
  - Decrease in concurrent medication affecting glycaemic control
  - Decrease in weight (particularly in elderly people)
  - Presence of renal failure

PATIENT AND CARER INFORMATION:
HYPOGLYCAEMIA PREVENTION

- Exercise, alcohol and sexual activity may lower your blood sugar (glucose) levels sufficiently to cause hypoglycaemia
- Eat regularly (meals and snacks). Do not delay or miss meals
- Make sure you have a healthy diet – check with the dietitian
- Remember to take recommended dose of medication
- Eat more starchy food if you increase your activity
- Anyone taking insulin should reduce the dose before strenuous activity
- Carry glucose tablets/sweets – always (keep some in the car when you are driving)
- CARRY IDENTIFICATION (NECKLACE, BRACELET OR CARD)

PATIENT AND CARER INFORMATION:
HYPOGLYCAEMIA MANAGEMENT

■ Recognise symptoms (sweating, trembling, confusion, etc) which may be special for you

■ Drink something sweet (fresh orange juice, Lucozade or Coca-Cola) or take six glucose tablets or eat a handful of sweets

■ If you are taking sulphonylureas, follow up your medication with a snack. Check your blood glucose to avoid over doing things

■ If you are driving:
   ◆ Slow down
   ◆ Stop the car safely
   ◆ Remove keys from the ignition
   ◆ Move to the passenger seat
   ◆ Treat the hypoglycaemia as above

■ Try to work out the cause of this hypoglycaemic attack:
   ◆ Too much insulin?
   ◆ Too little food?
   ◆ Delayed meal?
   ◆ More activity?
   ◆ Stress?
   ◆ Hot weather?
   ◆ New injection site used?

■ Be aware – there may be occasions when there is no apparent reason

HEART AND MAJOR VESSEL DISEASE

- Coronary heart disease (CHD) is much more common among people with diabetes and is the main cause of death (up to 75% in type 2 diabetes)

- Excess risk applies even to those with slightly raised blood glucose levels, ie fasting glucose > 6 mmol/l

- Type 2 diabetes increases the risk of myocardial infarct (MI) by 2–3 times

- The cardiac risk factors are cumulative

- Tight control of diabetes and blood pressure reduces the risk of CHD

- Patients with diabetes should stop smoking

- Maintain a high index of suspicion for cardiac disease in people with diabetes, even when they have no classic symptoms

- People with diabetes should have their cholesterol screened on diagnosis. If cardiovascular risk is >15%, take a statin, aiming to reduce cholesterol by 25% or to < 4 mmol/l, whichever is the greater

Stroke

- Stroke is more frequent in people with diabetes

- Multi-infarct dementia is also relatively common

- Prolonged or frequent hypoglycaemia can cause confusion, memory defects or paranoia in older people with diabetes, and may mimic a stroke or cerebrovascular disease

Lipids/cholesterol

- Targets: to keep low-density lipoprotein (LDL) cholesterol < 3.0 mmol/l, high-density lipoprotein (HDL) cholesterol > 1.2 mmol/l

- Treat people with diabetes as if they already have vascular disease
- Screen all those with diabetes on diagnosis, to achieve optimal control. Rescreen if control deteriorates or insulin is started
- Use a statin as first-line treatment. If triglycerides are also raised, consider a fibrate with or without a statin
- LDL is an important risk factor. Aim to lower this
- HDL is also an important risk factor. Aim to raise this if possible
- Total cholesterol of 4.0 mmol/l is a realistic target resulting in significant risk reduction

VITAL POINT

✱ Raised blood glucose and blood pressure are major risk factors for heart disease, stroke and peripheral circulatory problems

PATIENT AND CARER INFORMATION:
LOOKING AFTER YOUR HEART

- Diabetes increases the risk of a heart attack
- You should not smoke
- You should eat healthily – see a dietitian to check this out
- You should have your cholesterol checked on diagnosis of your diabetes
- You should have your cholesterol/lipids measured every year
- You should have regular blood pressure measurements and start treatment if it is raised
- Go to your GP urgently if you have any pain in your chest, arm or jaw, either at rest or on exercise
- Good control of blood sugar (glucose), blood pressure and cholesterol reduces the risk of heart disease and stroke

Peripheral vascular disease

- People with diabetes are 2–4 times more likely to develop intermittent claudication and 4–6 times more likely to have to undergo an amputation

- Screen all people with diabetes for peripheral vascular disease

- Ask about their smoking history and symptoms of intermittent claudication

- After 20 years of diabetes, 50% of men and 33% of women have no pulses in their feet

- At annual review, check patients' feet for ischaemia and feel for the pulses

- Refer to a vascular surgeon any patient with worsening symptoms or rest pain

- Critical ischaemia or gangrene requires urgent vascular referral

Peripheral neuropathy

- Evidence of neuropathy may be found in up to 50% of patients with type 2 diabetes, causing problems for about one-third of this population

- Lower limb and foot problems caused by peripheral neuropathy and ischaemia are common, causing prolonged hospital admission and amputation

- Identification of those at risk of foot ulceration, and educating these patients, are important preventive measures

Examination of the feet

With a little practice, a thorough foot examination can be carried out in a few minutes. All people with diabetes should have access to a state registered podiatrist. If there are any concerns, make a referral.

- Remove shoes and socks, tights or stockings

- Examine the patient lying on a couch or seated comfortably with both legs and feet raised

- Examine both feet for the following:
  - Condition of the skin (lower legs and feet)
  - Dry, flaky skin
  - Cracks or evidence of fungal infection between each toe (athlete's foot)
  - Colour of skin (lower legs and feet)
  - Corns, calluses, other deformities (on pressure-bearing points, eg tops of the toes)
  - Condition of toenails (whether thickened, long or horny)
  - Nail-cutting technique and/or evidence of ingrowing toenails
  - Discoloration or abnormal skin lesions
  - Evidence of infection (ie pain, lack of sensation, numbness, inflammation, cellulitis, exudate or swelling)
- Examine upper and lower surfaces of feet and toes (including heels)
- Record all abnormalities/changes
- Examine the feet for the dorsalis pedis and posterior tibial pulses
  - To check whether foot pulses are diminished, palpate popliteal and femoral pulses
  - Record changed, diminished or absent pulses
- Test sensation in feet:
  - Check sensation using a 10 g monofilament over the tips of the big and little toes and the base of the big toe (avoid callus)
  - Check vibration perception using a 128 Hz tuning fork and test big toe and medial malleolus
  - Test for motor neuropathy by looking for deformities in the toes and feet
  - Check knee and ankle jerks (with a tendon hammer)
  - Record defects in sensation
- Examine foot ulcers for inflammation and discharge (take swab for microbiology)
- Record and discuss foot problems with the patient as appropriate

Examination of footwear

- Shoes should be examined inside and outside, looking for evidence of the following:
  - General wear and tear
  - The need for repair
  - Gait change (one shoe more worn than the other)
  - Excessive weight bearing (heel or sole worn down)
  - Perforation of soles or heels (eg by nails)
  - Abrasive heels (especially with new shoes)
  - Damaging projections inside the shoes (causing pressure)
  - Worn insoles (causing pressure)
  - Poor fit of shoes (length and breadth)
- Problems identified with shoes should be recorded and discussed with the patient
- Socks, tights or stockings should be examined for:
  - The type of material (is it constricting – nylon or elasticated?)
  - Type of washing powder used (biological washing powders can be irritant)
  - The method of holding up socks (eg garters should not be used)
  - Presence and thickness of seams (these can cause traumatic ulcers)
- Problems identified should be recorded and discussed with the patient

Risk factors for foot ulcers

The following features put people at risk of foot ulcers:

- Living alone
- Drinking too much alcohol
- Poor eyesight
- Poor glycaemic control
- Poor self-image
- Living in a deprived area
- Other complications of diabetes
- Smoking cigarettes

- Male sex
- Walking or climbing in unaccustomed footwear

VITAL POINTS

* Emphasise to smokers that, as well as the better known consequences of smoking, they are also putting their feet at risk
* Examine the feet at least once a year
* Examine the feet to educate yourself and your patient
* Failure to do this may result in unnecessary amputations

PATIENT AND CARER INFORMATION:
LOOKING AFTER YOUR FEET

- Keep your feet clean: wash and dry gently between your toes
- Moisturise your feet (but not between your toes) with hand cream, olive oil or E45 cream. Do not dig down the sides of your toenails
- Cut your nails (softer after washing) according to the shape of your toes. If you cannot cut your own then request a visit to a state-registered chiropodist (podiatrist)
- Check your feet and shoes daily – using a mirror if necessary. You may not be aware of injuries
- If possible involve a third party, such as your partner
- Do not ignore even the slightest injury to your feet
- Report any sores, swelling, cracks, corns, skin damage or change of colour IMMEDIATELY to your doctor
- Avoid walking barefoot; you should wear shoes or slippers at all times
- Choose shoes that provide good support: broad, long and deep. Check that you can wriggle your toes inside your shoes. (As a general rule trainers are a good choice)

- Try to buy shoes where you can have them fitted by a trained person
- Wear new shoes for short periods of time to start with
- Check your shoes regularly for ridges, sharp points or nails; tip them out upside down before putting on
- Wear the correct shoes for the job and for the health of your feet
- Do not wear tight-fitting socks. Choose ones with no ridges if possible – if they have them, wear socks inside out
- Change socks or stockings/tights daily
- Avoid extremes of temperature, very hot baths, sitting close to fires and radiators, and hot water bottles
- Do not treat corns yourself. Visit a state-registered chiropodist
- Never use a surgical blade, corn-paring knife or corn remedies on your feet
- Treat your feet with respect

DIABETIC RETINOPATHY

Monitoring in primary care

- Check that the patient is visiting an optician annually, for visual acuity checks
- Arrange a retinal screening programme with photography
- If diabetic retinopathy is detected:
  - Give a gentle explanation of the problem – patients often find this information very frightening
  - Give information about the extent of retinal damage
  - If sight is threatened, ensure immediate referral to an ophthalmologist
  - Give support and reassurance because the individual will fear possible visual loss and treatment; there may be a bad family history of diabetic eye disease
  - Give information about laser therapy if required

- As chronic glaucoma is more common in people with diabetes, ensure that intraocular pressure is measured every year

- Ensure appropriate and timely referral to an ophthalmologist

- People with diabetes are more likely to develop cataracts; these must be treated early to allow the early detection of retinopathy. Arrange for an ophthalmological referral, so that cataract extraction can be undertaken at the optimal time

VITAL POINT

Ensure that all patients with type 2 diabetes have their retinas checked by an ophthalmologist or photographed every year

PATIENT AND CARER INFORMATION:

LOOKING AFTER YOUR EYES

General

- You must have your eyes checked once a year with eye drops, with a photograph of the retina (back of the eye)

- You are entitled to a free annual eye test if you take tablets or insulin, so take advantage of this!

- Ask your care team to explain what is being checked and what is happening

- If, on examination, you are found to have a condition called diabetic retinopathy, you will be referred to an ophthalmologist and may need laser therapy

- If so, ask for an information sheet about it

- Laser treatment may not improve your sight; but it prevents further deterioration

Laser therapy

- Laser therapy is given to prevent the progress of diabetic disease at the back of the eye (retina)

- Regular eye screening is important: ideally, you should be given laser therapy at an early stage before your sight has been affected

- The laser is a machine that produces a small spot of very bright light

- The light is so bright it produces a burn wherever it is focused

- Although the laser makes a burn in your eye, it is not usually painful because the retina cannot feel pain

- Sometimes, however, if you have had a lot of laser treatment, it may be uncomfortable and you will be offered a local anaesthetic

- Laser treatment is usually carried out in an outpatient department

- You will be able to go home after the treatment

- Your vision may be blurred or you may be dazzled by bright light (take dark glasses with you)

- You should not drive home after laser therapy, so it is best to make sure someone comes with you to the laser clinic

- After treatment, you may notice some reduction in your sight. This usually only lasts a few days. You may experience headaches

- As only one eye is treated at a time, if your other eye sees well your vision should not be too badly affected

- Most people do not need to take time off work after treatment

- You are required to declare on your driving licence application form that you have had laser treatment. You will probably need a visual fields test (to test the width of your vision)

- If you need large amounts of laser treatment, your field of vision may be affected

- Provided that you can read a number plate at 20.5 metres (67 feet) with or without spectacles, and you pass the visual fields test (as most people do) there will be no problem about your driving licence. You will need to adhere to the usual regulations for someone with diabetes

DIABETIC NEPHROPATHY

Monitoring in primary care

- Up to 40% of people with type 2 diabetes have some degree of renal disease
- There are four stages of diabetic renal disease:
  - Stage 1 or microalbuminuria (urine needs to be sent to the laboratory to detect microalbuminuria)
  - Stage 2 or albuminuria (detected in the clinic using Albustix)
  - Stage 3 or raised serum creatinine (once this is above the normal range, over half the normal kidney function has been lost)
  - Stage 4 or end-stage renal failure, requiring dialysis
- Delaying the progression of diabetic nephropathy involves three separate actions:
  - Aggressive control of blood pressure, which is nearly always raised
  - Tight blood glucose control
  - In type 1 diabetes, dietary protein restriction may be of benefit
- Established renal failure will require the following treatment options:
  - Haemodialysis
  - Continuous ambulatory peritoneal dialysis (CAPD)
  - Renal transplantation
- Check renal function 2 weeks after starting a patient on an ACE inhibitor or sartan

VITAL POINT

✷ Treat raised BP very aggressively in patients with kidney disease. This will postpone end-stage renal failure. Target systolic pressure is 130 mmHg

AUTONOMIC NEUROPATHY AND SEXUAL DYSFUNCTION

Monitoring in primary care

- Autonomic neuropathy affects 20–40% of all people with diabetes
- It may contribute to impotence in up to 50% of men with long-standing diabetes. Treatment for this condition is available
- It is often a 'hidden' problem, and may lead to marital difficulties
- Failure to gain an erection may be caused by:
  - Nerve damage
  - Poor circulation
  - Psychological factors
  - Drinking alcohol
  - Smoking and recreational drugs
  - Some treatments for high blood pressure or depression
- Treatment is available and is offered after assessment for possible causes. Treatments currently considered/offered are:
  - Counselling
  - Sildenafil and other drugs in the same group are available on prescription to men with diabetes and erection difficulties. These drugs are safe but should never be used by men taking a nitrate for their heart, which includes glyceryl trinitrate (GTN) tablets or spray for angina
  - Vacuum devices
  - Self-injection of alprostadil (Caverject, Viridal) into the penis
  - Penile implants (surgery)
- Refer to a specialist service if initial treatment fails

- Alcohol, smoking, recreational drugs and medication (for blood pressure or depression) can cause problems with erections
- You will have blood tests to check your diabetes control and hormone levels
- You could be referred to a specialist clinic
- There are various effective treatments:
  - Counselling
  - Injections
  - Vacuum devices
  - Surgery
  - Tablets
- Viagra (Sildenafil) and other drugs in the same group are available on prescription. Do not use if you are taking a nitrate for your heart. Beware of purchasing these drugs over the Internet as they may be fake

IMPACT OF THE MENOPAUSE:

RECOMMENDATIONS

- Postmenopausal women who have diabetes are no longer routinely advised to take hormone replacement therapy (HRT)
- HRT can increase breast cancer risk in some women so they will need to take part in a screening programme, as should all women over 50 according to national guidelines
- For women who also take insulin, starting HRT may require a small dose adjustment

10 How to manage type 1 diabetes

PRESENTATION AND DIAGNOSIS

- Diabetes care is a partnership between patients and professionals. However, at the onset, many patients will want the doctor and nurse to assume control. With time, patients gain in confidence and ownership of their diabetes

- Most people with type 1 diabetes are seen by a diabetes care team in secondary care, although they will occasionally present to the surgery

- Treat with insulin. Options for different insulin regimens should be discussed regularly. For up-to-date information, refer to British National Formulary or MIMS

- Basic lifestyle advice, such as NOT SMOKING, reduces the risks of heart disease, stroke and poor circulation

- People with type 1 diabetes feel more confident if they monitor their blood glucose levels several times a day, understand the results and take action on them

- The purpose of the monitoring is good glucose control, to keep people feeling well and to help to avoid both high and low blood glucose levels

- A range of blood glucose levels needs to be discussed. The ideal is 4–6 mmol/l before and < 9 mmol/l after a meal

- Patients must be aware of possible short- and long-term complications of their diabetes

- Regular visits and checks throughout the year provide opportunities for discussion and/or advice

- People with diabetes should expect an annual review:
  - Eye photograph
  - Foot inspection
  - Blood pressure check

- ◆ Urine tests for albumin and microalbuminuria
- ◆ Blood tests for cholesterol and creatinine
- ■ Advise that there can also be problems with good glucose control (weight gain, more severe hypos and less warning of a hypo). Help should be requested if any of these occur
- ■ People with diabetes need to find their own way of coping with diabetes in a way that suits their lifestyle

DOSE ADJUSTMENT FOR NORMAL EATING (DAFNE)

- ■ The DAFNE initiative is based on work pioneered in Germany and followed by a trial in the UK in 2000–2001
- ■ It involves educating patients to take control of their own diabetes and has been shown to be remarkably successful
- ■ So far, there are 37 DAFNE centres in the UK and Ireland, with a further 19 centres to be enrolled by February 2007
- ■ For where to find out more, see page 114

CHILDREN AND YOUNG PEOPLE: MAIN ISSUES

- ■ A child presenting with symptoms of diabetes needs immediate referral to hospital or a specialist diabetes centre for confirmation of diagnosis and assessment
- ■ The management plan should involve the primary care team
- ■ The primary care team must be kept advised of the child's health by the specialist team
- ■ You need to be prepared to talk with the child and family
- ■ Such children should receive the usual immunisations

- Children with diabetes often have wide fluctuations in their glucose control (especially if they are ill) and the primary care team needs to be able to deal with this

- When these children come to the surgery with other ailments, these should be considered in the light of their diabetes

- You should be available to provide extra support to the child and the family at difficult times such as changing school, puberty, etc

- The family may well need considerably more support than the average family

- Careful observation of relationships within the family is advisable. If necessary, be prepared to address these directly with the parents

VITAL POINT

* Make friends with your patients, and help them to accept their diabetes

11 How to manage pregnancy and gestational diabetes

PREGNANT WOMEN WITH DIABETES

- Any woman with diabetes contemplating pregnancy must have pre-pregnancy counselling with her partner
- All women planning a pregnancy should take a folic acid supplement
- Pregnancy complicates diabetes and diabetes complicates pregnancy
- Blood glucose control must be optimal (fasting levels between 4 and 6 mmol/l) before and throughout pregnancy to prevent complications/abnormalities in the baby and complications in the mother
- The woman needs to be aware of the risk of congenital abnormalities
- There are also risks to the woman herself – retinopathy and nephropathy may get worse
- The aim is normal delivery of baby but caesarean section is more likely (50%) if glucose control is poor
- Drugs cannot be used in pregnancy, so control has to be by diet and insulin. Those with type 2 diabetes have to start insulin, as drugs may harm the unborn baby
- A planned programme of care, with precise protocols, should be available to all the care teams and the mother. Diabetes specialist and obstetric teams should work in partnership
- Optimal blood glucose control increases the risk of hypoglycaemia
- Blood glucose should be monitored 4–6 times a day
- Insulin will need adjusting, often reaching two to three times the pre-pregnancy dose
- Diet should be controlled, with care about food intake and weight
- Overall good nutrition is essential
- Easy access to specialist nurses and midwives is vital

- All pregnant women with diabetes must visit the diabetic clinic at least every 4 weeks. HbAlc, blood pressure and urine albumin should be tested at every visit, eyes checked regularly, scans as agreed locally

- A planned delivery programme is needed

PRE-PREGNANCY AND FAMILY PLANNING ADVICE

- Ask for advice about pregnancy well before you plan to have children

- If you want to start a pregnancy you should eat a good, balanced diet and take a folic acid supplement

- Discuss with your doctor what your target blood sugar levels should be before conceiving, and how best to maintain them

- The contraceptive pill does not suit everybody. It may carry extra risks if you are older, overweight or smoke, or if you have high blood pressure or a tendency to blood clots

- Low-dose combined contraceptive pills do not usually have any effects on diabetes, but you should check your blood glucose levels and have regular blood pressure tests

- Low-dose progestogen-only pills are safe in diabetes, but are less reliable than the low-dose combined pill

- You can use the coil (IUD) or barrier methods (caps and condoms). If you do not plan to have more children, you can be sterilised or your partner can have a vasectomy

GESTATIONAL DIABETES MELLITUS (GDM)

- This is diabetes that starts/occurs only during pregnancy
- If fasting blood glucose is borderline, confirm the diagnosis by an oral glucose tolerance test
- Protocols for identifying GDM vary throughout the country. Use the local one
- Refer the woman to a specialist diabetes team
- If diabetes presents late in pregnancy, it may have been hidden throughout the pregnancy. Urgent referral is required
- Pregnant women have a lower renal threshold so glycosuria is not diagnostic of gestational diabetes
- Management is by diet and monitoring of weight. Insulin may be required
- If blood glucose levels are not kept within range by diet (< 6 mmol/l before meals and < 8 mmol/l after), insulin treatment will be necessary
- Frequent blood glucose monitoring is essential – before and 2 hours after meals
- Women should have a glucose tolerance test at 6-week postnatal visit and IGT or IFG are both common
- Gestational diabetes carries a 50% risk of type 2 diabetes later in life
- Women with gestational diabetes need to be informed of this problem and counselled about maintaining a healthy lifestyle to reduce the risk of type 2 diabetes: plenty of exercise and weight control
- They need lifelong monitoring for diabetes – usually an annual fasting blood glucose test

VITAL POINTS

* Early referral to obstetric diabetes service is essential
* 50% of women with gestational diabetes will develop type 2 diabetes in later life

12 Living with diabetes

Living with diabetes means looking after yourself – not just the control of blood sugar (glucose), but also your feet, eyes, teeth (dentist) and making sure you are up to date with your immunisations. In other words it is looking after your health generally. There are also certain areas where you will have to be particularly careful (such as family planning – see page 85 – or travelling). You also need to be aware of possible legal restrictions (regarding driving, for example).

PATIENT AND CARER INFORMATION:

IMMUNISATION

- All routine immunisations are safe for you

- If you are travelling abroad, check with your GP whether further immunisations are needed

- If you are aged over 65, you should have a 'flu immunisation: this should be available during October/November each year

- Pneumococcal immunisation is available to anyone over 2 years of age with diabetes; it can be given with the influenza immunisation

- Immunisation can have an effect on your diabetes; test your sugar (glucose) levels more frequently and if necessary increase your dose of insulin or tablets

---

PATIENT AND CARER INFORMATION:
DENTAL CARE

- Make sure your dentist knows you have diabetes
- Go for regular check-ups
- Get early treatment for infections as they may upset your glucose control
- General anaesthetics should be carried out in hospital
- A painful mouth can cause low blood glucose levels if eating is affected
- You will not receive any special financial help with dental fees

PATIENT AND CARER INFORMATION:
LIFE INSURANCE

- Life insurance is calculated according to age and state of health and likelihood of survival
- A life insurance policy already held should not be affected by the diagnosis of diabetes. It is not necessary to declare your diabetes once a policy has been agreed
- If a new policy is taken out, your diabetes must be declared and the policy may be loaded. This can be challenged
- Advice about helpful insurance companies can be obtained from Diabetes UK (tel: 0800 731 7431)

- Car driving licences can be held by people with diabetes

- Those treated with diet alone or tablets are not subject to licence restrictions (for diabetes). They can retain their 'until aged 70' privilege, but must inform the DVLA of any treatment change

- Licences are renewed every 1, 2 or 3 years depending on health (of people treated with insulin)

- The DVLA (see page 115) must be told of your diabetes and any treatment change (eg from diet alone to tablets or tablets to insulin), unless diabetes is diet controlled. This is required by law. NOTE: this information must be provided and recorded. The decision to follow this advice is the responsibility of the individual concerned

- Licence renewal forms are sent automatically before the expiry date. There is no fee for renewal

- Licence renewal is granted after completion of the form by the person with diabetes (including signed consent for the individual's doctor to be consulted by the DVLA, if required)

- A medical check may be requested by the DVLA

- The driver must inform his or her driving insurance company of the presence of diabetes

- Insurance companies may load the driver's premium. This should be challenged and it is sensible to 'shop around' because the Disability Discrimination Act 1995 has helped this situation

- Diabetes UK Services (see page 115) can also offer motor insurance cover

PATIENT AND CARER INFORMATION:
OCCUPATIONAL LICENCES

■ People whose diabetes is treated by diet alone, or diet and tablets, are normally allowed to hold LGV (large goods vehicle) and PCV (passenger carrying vehicle) licences, provided they are otherwise in good health

■ People treated with insulin are not allowed to hold these licences

■ Anyone who starts using insulin must inform the DVLA and stop driving the vehicle immediately

■ Patients taking insulin may be able to apply for a licence to drive vehicles weighing 3.5–7.5 tonnes (category C1) provided they fulfil a number of strict medical conditions

■ The law does not bar insulin-users from driving taxis (provided there are fewer than nine seats). However, many local taxi licensing authorities do apply blanket restrictions

- You may require immunisation, which could affect your blood glucose control

- Travel insurance needs to include adequate cover, including for your diabetes. Contact Diabetes UK for information (tel: 020 7424 1000)

- Obtain a European Health Insurance Card from your surgery, or you can apply for one online at www.dh.gov.uk/travellers

- This website provides information on travelling and health, and medical care in the European Community

- Take with you:
  - Identification
  - A letter from your doctor
  - Medication for travel sickness and diarrhoea
  - Antibiotics
  - Simple dressings
  - An adequate supply of diabetes medication
  - Sunscreen (at least factor 15)
  - Appropriate footwear
  - Sweets or biscuits for travel

- If you are treated with insulin, take testing equipment and a cool bag. Keep your supplies in the cool bag and carry it with your hand luggage

- With the heightened security that often operates in today's airports, it is a wise precaution to carry a letter from your doctor stating that you have diabetes and need insulin injections or other medication

EMERGENCIES

The following situations require **immediate** referral to hospital:

- A person with severe hypoglycaemia who is not responding to glucagon
- A person with possible ketoacidosis (unwell with ketones)
- A person with newly diagnosed type 1 diabetes and severe symptoms
- A person with newly diagnosed type 2 diabetes and severe symptoms
- A child diagnosed with diabetes
- A person (particularly an older person) with diabetes who is severely dehydrated (hyperosmolar coma)
- Anyone with a diabetic foot ulcer that gets markedly worse (eg any change in colour, new onset of pain, redness or swelling)
- Anyone with diabetes who experiences a sudden deterioration in their sight (eg retinal haemorrage/retinal detachment)

Ketoacidosis

- Ketoacidosis is the most common cause of death in people with diabetes aged under 20. This may result from delaying treatment in patients with ketoacidosis
- If ketoacidosis develops, refer the patient straight to hospital. Suspect if unwell, particularly if there is abdominal pain, vomiting or shortness of breath
- Intravenous fluids are needed
- Blood glucose levels should be closely monitored
- Ketoacidosis may result from delay in diagnosing type 1 diabetes and from wrong medical advice (eg incorrect instructions to stop insulin during intercurrent illness)

- The correct advice is to KEEP testing blood glucose and taking insulin. Insulin may need to be increased, depending on the results of the blood glucose tests

Monitoring in primary care

- Monitoring equipment such as Ketostix and blood glucose test strips (in date and kept in airtight containers in a dry place, not in a fridge) should be available in the surgery and doctor's bag

- Short-acting insulin may be useful to lower blood glucose levels in acute illness (in the surgery and doctor's bag)

- Review therapy and treat intercurrent illness

- Consider short-term insulin therapy

- Vomiting with either hyperglycaemia or ketoacidosis is a medical emergency. It requires immediate hospital admission for intravenous insulin and fluids

- Blood glucose control may deteriorate rapidly during an illness of any kind. Teach people with diabetes when they need to get help

- Also teach the relative or carer, in case the person with diabetes is too unwell to look after themselves

- For those with type 2 diabetes on insulin, if possible and appropriate, teach the relative or carer to draw up and give insulin if necessary and to monitor blood glucose levels

- Give an emergency contact telephone number to the person with diabetes and/or a relative

- Glucagon is necessary for treatment of severe hypoglycaemia. You must show a relative/carer how to use it

* For people with diabetes, vomiting is a danger sign and needs urgent action

PATIENT AND CARER INFORMATION:

WHAT TO DO WHEN YOU'RE ILL

- A minor illness, such as a cold, may cause your blood glucose levels to rise
- Keep taking your tablets (or insulin) even if you are not eating
- Blood glucose levels will return to normal once the infection is over
- Consult your doctor if the illness persists or if you have high blood test results
- Headaches and sore throats can be safely treated with paracetamol or aspirin
- Sugar-free cough remedies are available from your local pharmacist
- Vomiting may prevent you from keeping down tablets – consult your doctor
- Vomiting and diarrhoea may cause serious loss of fluid – you need urgent medical help
- This fluid may need to be replaced by means of a drip
- Even if your diabetes is normally controlled by tablets, you may need insulin for a time

IMPORTANT RULES

- Continue taking your diabetes treatment (diet and tablets or insulin)
- Make sure you drink plenty of liquid (water, tea, etc)
- Test your urine or blood every day to check your progress
- If you are not hungry, substitute meals with a liquid or light diet (soup, ice cream, glucose drinks, milk)
- Consult your doctor in good time. It is a medical emergency if you are vomiting and unable to keep down fluids

PRACTICE AND SHARED PROTOCOLS

- Your PCT should have agreed protocols with secondary care in line with the NSF (see Appendix 2)

- The GP contract (see below and Appendix 3) is designed to force down the targets for cardiovascular risk factors

- There needs to be an ongoing clinical audit of practice-based diabetes services. Select the criteria and agree standards of care for audit

- Anonymous data from district, regional and national groups enable evaluation of effectiveness

- In the short term, monitor:
  - ◆ The process of care
  - ◆ The prevalence of cardiovascular risk factors
  - ◆ Markers of late complications
  - ◆ Acute and intermediate outcomes

- It is valuable to collate data at a local level on a district diabetes register

AUDIT AND QUALITY CONTROL MONITORING

The GMS GP Contract

- The GP Contract aims to reward practices on the quality of care delivered to patients

- Indicators are used to assess the quality of care provided, by awarding points for meeting targets in different areas of performance. Because they come with funding, they are likely to be the drivers for clinical care

- In the clinical domain, the Contract focuses on ten key areas, including coronary heart disease, stroke, hypertension and diabetes

- There are 18 clinical indicators relating to diabetes (see Appendix 3)
- There is an emphasis on helping patients give up smoking
- The remaining targets are clinical and some patients may find them hard to achieve. They are designed to put downward pressure on cardio-vascular risk factors such as HbA1c, blood pressure and cholesterol
- There are (financial) points for the following process measures:
  - BMI
  - HbA1c
  - Screening for retinopathy
  - Neuropathy and peripheral vascular disease
  - Microalbuminuria
  - Checking serum cholesterol, serum creatinine and blood pressure
- Targets for clinical outcomes are HbA1c <7.4%, BP <145/85 mmg and total cholesterol <5.0 mmol/l

Process measures

- For the majority of patients with type 2 diabetes, the process and outcome measures prescribed by the GP contract will become standard
- Apart from clinic measures, there are three other domains in the quality framework:
  - Organisational (including training and education)
  - Additional services
  - Patient experience. This consists of patient surveys and will encourage practices to measure patient satisfaction

Serious complications of diabetes

So far the GP contract does not address the serious complications of diabetes and these should be part of a practice audit. They include the following:

- Patients with nephropathy (microalbuminuria, proteinuria or raised serum creatinine)
- Patients who have needed laser therapy or vitrectomy for diabetic retinopathy
- Patients with cataract, background or sight-threatening retinopathy
- Patients with visual impairment

- Patients with absent foot pulses (see foot risk score – Appendix 2)
- Patients with reduced vibration sense (see foot risk score – Appendix 2)
- Patients with foot ulceration (previous or present)
- Patients with symptomatic neuropathy
- Male patients with erectile dysfunction
- Patients with angina
- Patients with claudication
- Patients who have had myocardial infarction
- Patients who have had a stroke
- Patients with end-stage renal failure
- Patients who have had a major amputation (above the ankle) or minor amputation (below the ankle)
- Age-specific mortality in people with diabetes
- Outcomes of pregnancies in women with pre-existing or gestational diabetes:
  - Birth rates
  - Abortion rates: spontaneous and terminations
  - Stillbirth rates and peri-neonatal mortality rates
  - Incidence of congenital abnormalities

THE PRIMARY HEALTH CARE TEAM

People with diabetes receive the best care when there is a strong diabetes team in their practice. The key members are the GP and practice nurse(s). Apart from the patient and carer, the team needs support from a dietitian, a podiatrist and a pharmacist.

General practitioners

Each practice needs a dedicated GP for diabetes with the following roles:

- With the diabetes nurse, to plan the structure of care
- To set up an effective practice register of diabetes
- To map a care pathway for newly diagnosed patients

- To examine educational and training issues
- To audit results in the light of the GMS GP Contract (see pages 95–7 and Appendix 3)

Nurses

One or more practice nurses should take the lead for diabetes, and be responsible for the following:

- Working with the GP to plan care for diabetes
- Becoming an expert resource for patients with diabetes
- Forging links with specialist nurses in secondary care

Pharmacists

- Pharmacists are a regular point of contact for people with diabetes and can play a central role in improved medicines management
- The Department of Health has already published medicines management guidance as part of the NSF for older people
- It is now developing guidance for medicines management in long-term conditions, supporting the NSFs for diabetes, renal services and long-term conditions. This will be available soon

Dietitians

- In some parts of the UK, dietitians are thin on the ground
- They have a vital role in planning educational care for patients and training other health care professionals in dietetics

Podiatrists

- Specialist podiatry services are becoming more established in the UK. They have the following roles:
  - Providing training for other professionals
  - Setting up a system for screening patients for foot problems
  - Offering a rapid access service for acute foot problems

The patient and family

- The patient is a very important part of the team, and may well know more about his or her diabetes than anyone else
- Involve the patient and carer/family wherever possible

Appendix 1
Self-monitoring: blood glucose and urine

- Urine testing is appropriate in situations where:
  - ◆ Blood glucose monitoring is not possible
  - ◆ Or the patient has a preference not to blood test

- HbA1c target = below 7.5%

- Increase testing frequency during:
  - ◆ Pregnancy
  - ◆ Times of illness
  - ◆ Changes in therapy
  - ◆ Changes in routine
  - ◆ Times of poor control
  - ◆ When at risk of hypoglycaemia
  - ◆ (Also if hypoglycaemia is a problem, especially when driving)

Blood glucose monitoring targets

Fasting	4–7 mmol/l	Bedtime	5–10 mmol/l
Pre-prandial	4–7 mmol/l	Post-prandial	< 11 mmol/l

- Self-monitoring does not replace regular HbA1c testing, which remains the gold standard test, and should only be used in conjunction with appropriate therapy as part of integrated care

Blood glucose self-monitoring guidelines

Education and lifestyle interventions	■ Advice on diet, exercise and smoking habit, key interventions at diagnosis and beyond ■ If necessary, patients should receive education relevant to **appropriate** testing, **understanding when** to test and what to do with the result	All patients who are self-monitoring should be encouraged to use the minimum number of tests required to keep control	
Newly diagnosed type 2 patient + diet control only Recommended regimen **A**	■ Self-monitoring may be required at diagnosis or as necessary depending on overall diabetic control and management plan ■ Self-monitoring may not be necessary if control is acceptable (eg HbA1c to target) ■ Health care professional should advise patient when self-monitoring becomes necessary	Urine testing may be appropriate for some patients in this group provided HbA1c targets are achieved	Typical weekly strip usage **0–6**
Type 2 patient prescribed oral therapy Recommended regimens **A B C**	■ Re-assess patient need and educate prior to initiation of single oral therapy or combined treatment ■ If self-monitoring is necessary, the health care professional should tailor monitoring regimen to individual patient need, depending on diabetic control ■ Special focus on testing to prevent hypoglycaemia, especially in sulpho-nylurea therapy	If starting self-monitoring at this stage teach patient before initiating new therapy	Typical weekly strip usage **0–14**
Type 2 patient prescribed insulin Recommended regimens **B D E**	■ Self-monitoring is recommended in all cases with daily testing on initiation of insulin ■ Once a patient is stable, frequency of profiles can be reduced to profiles on 1–2 days a week or daily at varying times (week profile)	Stable patients are those whose blood glucose varies little from day to day and who are not having intensive changes of treatment	Typical weekly strip usage **4–28**

Blood glucose self-monitoring guidelines (cont'd)

Type 1 patients Recommended regimens **E F**	■ Self-monitoring is strongly recommended in all cases ■ Self-monitoring should be used to adjust insulin dose before meals where this appropriate (eg Basal-Bolus regimen, pump therapy) ■ Self-monitoring in type 1 diabetes may only be required on 1–2 days per week in stable patients and depending on patient's daily routine	Typical weekly strip usage **8–28**

Examples of typical self-monitoring regimens

Regimen	**A**	One or two tests a week
Regimen	**B**	Once daily at various times (Week profile)
Regimen	**C**	Two tests daily
Regimen	**D**	Four tests at different times on one day (Day profile)
Regimen	**E**	Day profile twice a week
Regimen	**F**	Test before meals and at bedtime each day

Appendix 2
Specimen agreed protocols
with secondary care

Guidelines for management of type 2 diabetes from diagnosis

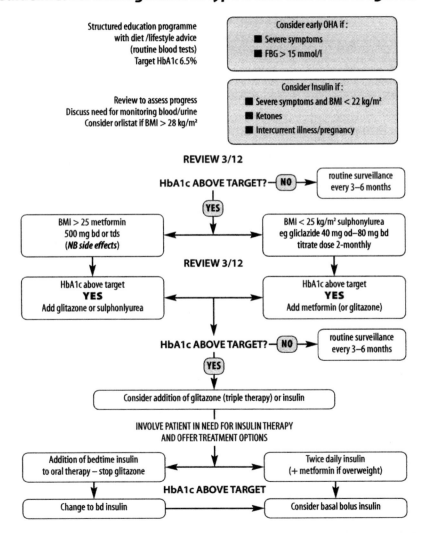

Structured education programme
with diet /lifestyle advice
(routine blood tests)
Target HbA1c 6.5%

Consider early OHA if :
- Severe symptoms
- FBG > 15 mmol/l

Review to assess progress
Discuss need for monitoring blood/urine
Consider orlistat if BMI > 28 kg/m²

Consider Insulin if :
- Severe symptoms and BMI < 22 kg/m²
- Ketones
- Intercurrent illness/pregnancy

REVIEW 3/12

HbA1c ABOVE TARGET? — NO → routine surveillance every 3–6 months

YES

BMI > 25 metformin
500 mg bd or tds
(*NB side effects*)

BMI < 25 kg/m² sulphonylurea
eg gliclazide 40 mg od–80 mg bd
titrate dose 2-monthly

REVIEW 3/12

HbA1c above target
YES
Add glitazone or sulphonlyurea

HbA1c above target
YES
Add metformin (or glitazone)

HbA1c ABOVE TARGET? — NO → routine surveillance every 3–6 months

YES

Consider addition of glitazone (triple therapy) or insulin

INVOLVE PATIENT IN NEED FOR INSULIN THERAPY
AND OFFER TREATMENT OPTIONS

Addition of bedtime insulin
to oral therapy – stop glitazone

Twice daily insulin
(+ metformin if overweight)

HbA1c ABOVE TARGET

Change to bd insulin

Consider basal bolus insulin

Diabetes guidelines: blood pressure management

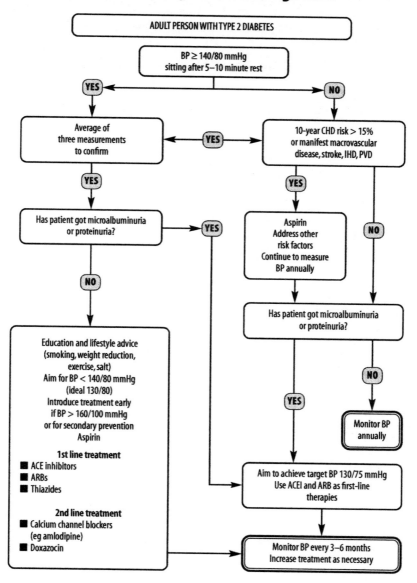

ADULT PERSON WITH TYPE 2 DIABETES

BP ≥ 140/80 mmHg
sitting after 5–10 minute rest

YES / **NO**

Average of
three measurements
to confirm

YES

10-year CHD risk > 15%
or manifest macrovascular
disease, stroke, IHD, PVD

YES

Has patient got microalbuminuria
or proteinuria?

YES

NO

Aspirin
Address other
risk factors
Continue to measure
BP annually

NO

Has patient got microalbuminuria
or proteinuria?

NO

Education and lifestyle advice
(smoking, weight reduction,
exercise, salt)
Aim for BP < 140/80 mmHg
(ideal 130/80)
Introduce treatment early
if BP > 160/100 mmHg
or for secondary prevention
Aspirin

1st line treatment
■ ACE inhibitors
■ ARBs
■ Thiazides

2nd line treatment
■ Calcium channel blockers
(eg amlodipine)
■ Doxazocin

YES

Monitor BP
annually

Aim to achieve target BP 130/75 mmHg
Use ACEI and ARB as first-line
therapies

Monitor BP every 3–6 months
Increase treatment as necessary

Diabetes guidelines: lipids

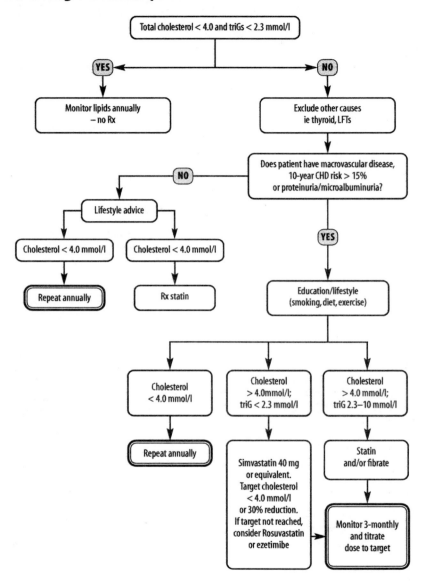

Total cholesterol < 4.0 and triGs < 2.3 mmol/l

YES → Monitor lipids annually – no Rx

NO → Exclude other causes ie thyroid, LFTs

Does patient have macrovascular disease, 10-year CHD risk > 15% or proteinuria/microalbuminuria?

NO → Lifestyle advice
- Cholesterol < 4.0 mmol/l → Repeat annually
- Cholesterol < 4.0 mmol/l → Rx statin

YES → Education/lifestyle (smoking, diet, exercise)

- Cholesterol < 4.0 mmol/l → Repeat annually
- Cholesterol > 4.0mmol/l; triG < 2.3 mmol/l → Simvastatin 40 mg or equivalent. Target cholesterol < 4.0 mmol/l or 30% reduction. If target not reached, consider Rosuvastatin or ezetimibe
- Cholesterol > 4.0 mmol/l; triG 2.3–10 mmol/l → Statin and/or fibrate → Monitor 3-monthly and titrate dose to target

Diabetes guidelines: feet

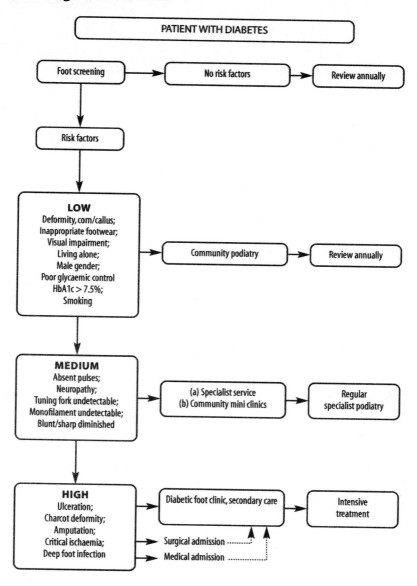

PATIENT WITH DIABETES

Foot screening → No risk factors → Review annually

Risk factors

LOW
Deformity, corn/callus;
Inappropriate footwear;
Visual impairment;
Living alone;
Male gender;
Poor glycaemic control
HbA1c > 7.5%;
Smoking

→ Community podiatry → Review annually

MEDIUM
Absent pulses;
Neuropathy;
Tuning fork undetectable;
Monofilament undetectable;
Blunt/sharp diminished

→ (a) Specialist service
(b) Community mini clinics → Regular specialist podiatry

HIGH
Ulceration;
Charcot deformity;
Amputation;
Critical ischaemia;
Deep foot infection

→ Diabetic foot clinic, secondary care → Intensive treatment
→ Surgical admission ....
→ Medical admission ....

Appendix 3
The GMS GP Contract:
Clinical Quality indicators for diabetes

Indicator	Points	Maximum threshold
Records		
DM 1: The practice can produce a register of all patients with diabetes mellitus	6	
Ongoing Management		
DM 2: The percentage of patients with diabetes whose notes record BMI in the previous 15 months	3	90%
DM 3: The percentage of patients with diabetes in whom there is a record of smoking status in the previous 15 months except those who have never smoked where smoking status should be recorded once	3	90%
DM 4: The percentage of patients with diabetes who smoke and whose notes contain a record that smoking cessation advice has been offered in the last 15 months	5	90%
DM 5: The percentage of diabetic patients who have a record of HbA1c or equivalent in the previous 15 months	3	90%
DM 6: The percentage of patients with diabetes in whom the last HbA1c is 7.4 or less (or equivalent test / reference range depending on local laboratory) in last 15 months	16	50%
DM 7: The percentage of patients with diabetes in whom the last HbA1c is 10 or less (or equivalent test / reference range depending on local laboratory) in last 15 months	11	85%
DM 8: The percentage of patients with diabetes who have a record of retinal screening in the previous 15 months	5	90%
DM 9: The percentage of patients with diabetes with a record of presence or absence of peripheral pulses in the previous 15 months	3	90%

Indicator		Points	Maximum threshold
	Ongoing Management		
DM 10:	The percentage of patients with diabetes with a record of neuropathy testing in the previous 15 months	3	90%
DM 11:	The percentage of patients with diabetes who have a record of the blood pressure in the past 15 months	3	90%
DM 12:	The percentage of patients with diabetes in whom the last blood pressure is 145/85 mmHg or less	17	55%
DM 13:	The percentage of patients with diabetes who have a record of microalbuminuria testing in the previous 15 months (exception reporting for patients with proteinuria)	3	90%
DM 14:	The percentage of patients with diabetes who have a record of serum creatinine testing in the previous 15 months	3	90%
DM 15:	The percentage of patients with diabetes with proteinuria or microalbuminuria who are treated with ACE inhibitors (or A2 antagonists)	3	70%
DM 16:	The percentage of patients with diabetes who have a record of total cholesterol in the previous 15 months	3	90%
DM 17:	The percentage of patients with diabetes whose last measured total cholesterol within previous 15 months is 5 or less	6	60%
DM 18:	The percentage of patients with diabetes who have had influenza immunisation in the preceding 1 September to 31 August	3	85%

Glossary of terms

ACE inhibitor: a class of drugs whose names end in 'pril', used in hypertension and cardiac failure. They are thought to protect the kidneys in early nephropathy

albuminuria: the presence of albumin in the urine denotes a urinary infection or kidney damage

Alpha cells: cells found in the pancreas which produce glucagon

AT2 blockers: angiotensin 2 blockers, also called angiotensin receptor blockers (ARBs) or sartans. Similar in action to ACE inhibitors. Possibly more effective in protecting kidneys. Cause less problem with cough

ARBs: see AT2 blockers

autonomic neuropathy: damage to the system of nerves that regulate many autonomic functions of the body such as stomach emptying, sexual function (potency), heart rate and blood pressure control

beta blockers: drugs that block the effect of stress hormones on the cardiovascular system. Often used to treat angina and raised blood pressure. They do not change the warning signs of hypoglycaemia or worsen peripheral vascular disease

beta cell (ß cell): the cell that produces insulin, found in the islets of Langerhans within the pancreas

biguanides: a group of tablets that lower blood glucose levels. The only one in use is metformin

blood glucose monitoring: system of measuring blood glucose levels at home using special reagent sticks and a meter

body mass index (BMI): body weight corrected for height expressed as weight in kg/(height in metres)^2. A normal BMI is 20–25 kgm^2

diabetes mellitus: a disorder of the pancreas characterised by a high blood glucose level

Diabetes UK: formerly known as the British Diabetic Association (BDA). Founded in 1938 by RD Lawrence, the foremost doctor specialising in diabetes, and HG Wells, the famous author. Both had diabetes and Diabetes UK has maintained the valuable collaboration between people with diabetes and health care professionals

diabetic coma: extreme form of hyperglycaemia, usually with ketoacidosis, causing unconsciousness

diabetic nephropathy: kidney damage caused by diabetes

diabetic neuropathy: nerve damage caused by diabetes

diabetic retinopathy: retinal damage caused by diabetes

dietary fibre: part of plant material that resists digestion and gives bulk to the diet. Also called fibre or roughage

diuretics: drugs that increase the volume of urine – usually called water tablets

fructosamine: measurement of glucose control, similar to HbA1c; it reflects average blood sugar (glucose) over previous 2–3 weeks. Cheaper but less reliable than HbA1c

gestational diabetes mellitus (GDM): diabetes occurring during pregnancy, with recovery after delivery

glaucoma: disease of the eye causing increased pressure inside the eyeball

glitazones: drugs (also called thiazolidinediones or PPAR-gamma agonists) that reduce blood glucose and insulin levels. They reduce insulin resistance, making the available insulin more effective. They also have effects on a range of risk factors

glucagon: a hormone which can be injected to increase blood glucose level. Used in severe hypos

glycosuria: presence of glucose in the urine

HbA1c (glycated haemoglobin): the part of the haemoglobin that has glucose attached to it. The percentage depends on the average blood glucose level over the previous 2–3 months

hyperglycaemia: high blood glucose (> 12 mmol/l)

hyperlipidaemia: an excess of fats (or lipids) in the blood

hypoglycaemia (also known as a hypo or an insulin reaction): low blood glucose (< 3.5 mmol/l)

impaired fasting glycaemia (IFG): a new category, which includes people with fasting glucose levels above normal, but not enough to diagnose diabetes, ie between 6.1 and 7.0 mmol/l

impaired glucose tolerance (IGT): is defined by a 2-hour glucose during an OGTT of > 7.8 mmol/l, but < 11.1 mmol/l plus a fasting plasma glucose < 7.0 mmol/l

insulin resistance: condition in which higher concentrations of insulin are required to achieve the same biological effect

islets of Langerhans: specialised cells within the pancreas that produce insulin and glucagon

ketoacidosis: a serious condition caused by lack of insulin and high blood glucose levels which results in body fat being used up to form ketones and acids. Characterised by high blood glucose levels, ketones in the urine, vomiting, drowsiness, heavy laboured breathing and a smell of acetone on the breath

ketonuria: the presence of acetone and other ketones in the urine. Detected by testing with a special testing stick (Ketostix,Ketur Test) or tablet (Acetest). Presence of ketones in the urine is due to lack of insulin. Small amounts of ketones may result from fasting, especially in children

laser treatment: process in which laser beams are used to treat a damaged retina (back of the eye).Widely used in diabetic retinopathy

metabolic syndrome: a cluster of medical problems – diabetes, hypertension, central obesity, abnormal lipids, coronary heart disease – all linked to insulin resistance. Also known as insulin resistance syndrome, Reaven's syndrome or syndrome X

microalbuminuria: excretion of traces of protein in the urine; an indication of early and treatable renal disease. Also a marker of macrovascular complications

National Service Framework (NSF): A government initiative designed to improve the quality of care for people with diabetes, regardless of where they live or who they are

nephropathy: kidney damage. In the first instance this makes the kidney leak so that small amounts of albumin appear in the urine. At a later stage it may affect the function of the kidney and in severe cases lead to kidney failure

NICE: The National Institute for Health and Clinical Excellence is a government body which aims to set standards for patients in the National Health Service. NICE makes recommendations on treatments and care using the best available evidence, and has produced a number of clinical guidelines relating to diabetes

neuropathy: damage to the nerves, either peripheral or autonomic or both. Occurs in diabetes

oral glucose tolerance test (OGTT): blood glucose is measured fasting and 2 hours after 75 g glucose syrup

peripheral neuropathy: damage to the nerves supplying the muscles and skin. May result in diminished sensation, muscle wasting and/or pain, particularly in the feet and legs

polydipsia: excessive thirst and drinking. A symptom of untreated diabetes and a high blood glucose

polyuria: the passing of large quantities of urine as a result of excess glucose in the bloodstream. Leads to polydipsia

postprandial glucose regulators: drugs that reduce blood glucose levels with a similar mode of action to sulphonylureas, but with a faster onset and shorter duration of action. Also called insulin secretagogues

PPAR-gamma agonists: drugs (also called thiazolidinediones or glitazones) that reduce blood glucose and insulin levels. They improve insulin resistance, resulting in increased effectiveness of available insulin

proteinuria: protein or albumin in the urine. A sign of nephropathy or urinary infection.

retinopathy: damage to the retina

sulphonylureas: tablets that lower the blood glucose by stimulating the pancreas to produce more insulin. Commonly used sulphonylureas are glibenclamide, gliclazide, glipizide and glimepiride

thiazolidinediones: drugs (also called PPAR-gamma agonists or glitazones) that reduce blood glucose and insulin levels. They reduce insulin resistance, resulting in increased effectiveness of available insulin

type 1 diabetes: refers to young people (usually < 40 years), who usually develop diabetes over a short space of time and always need insulin. Previously called insulin-dependent diabetes (IDDM)

type 2 diabetes: most common form of diabetes (80%), which usually develops in middle age but is becoming increasingly common in young people. It initially responds to diet and/or tablets but most people end up needing insulin. Previously called non insulin-dependent diabetes (NIDDM)

UK Prospective Diabetes Study (UKPDS): a study designed to answer the question of whether tight control of blood glucose and blood pressure influenced the outcome of type 2 diabetes. The results, published in September 1998, suggested that tight control of both factors lead to positive benefits in reducing the risk of diabetic complications

Resources

SELF-HELP FOR THE PRIMARY CARE TEAM

- Organise your own education by attending courses/conferences
- Find a 'buddy' practice to befriend and learn and share experiences
- Locate a 'mentor' practice with long experience of provision of diabetes care
- Contact the hospital-based local diabetes team and request resources and education
- Contact Diabetes UK for further information (see page 115)
- Driving and diabetes: see the Diabetes UK leaflet (see page 115)
- Join Diabetes UK (diabetes.org.uk)

Mainly for general practitioners

- Postgraduate Course in Diabetes held annually – changing centres every 2–3 years. Details from specialist diabetes physicians or Diabetes UK
- Local initiatives – through General Practitioner Training Schemes. Postgraduate Centres, RCGP Training, Diabetes Team Initiatives (PGEA schemes usually sought)
- The Primary Care Training Centre in Bradford run a 6-month course for health professionals currently working with patients who have diabetes. For more details, ring 01274 617617, or email: admin@primarycaretraining.co.uk
- Warwick Diabetes Care (University of Warwick) – a coherent point of contact for providers of diabetes care in the following ways: providing and promoting multidisciplinary diabetes education courses for health care professionals; undertaking and supporting applied diabetes research; developing practical resources and networks. For more details, ring 024 7657 2958 or email: diabetes@warwick.ac.uk

USEFUL REPORTS/KEY REFERENCES

Alberti KGMM (1999) The diagnosis and classification of diabetes mellitus. *Diabetes Voice* 44: 35–41

Anglo-Scandinavian Cardiac Outcomes Trial (ASCOT) Full information on results and publications can be found on the study website: www.ascotstudy.org

Audit Commission National Report (2000) *Test Times – a review of diabetes services in England and Wales*. Oxon: Audit Commission Publications

Budd S, Gatling W, Currell I, Mullee MA (1998) The Poole Diabetes Study: the prevalence of diagnosed diabetes mellitus in an English community in 1996. *Diabetes Today* 1: 12–4

CARDS investigators (2004) Primary prevention of cardiovascular disease with atorvastatin in type 2 diabetes in the Collaborative Atorvastatin Diabetes Study (CARDS): multicentre randomised placebo-controlled trial. *Lancet*, Aug 21, 364 (9435): 641–2

Department of Health (2001) *National Service Framework for Diabetes: Standards*. London: Department of Health

Department of Health (2002) *National Service Framework for Diabetes: Implementation*. London: Department of Health

Gerstein HC, Yusuf S, Bosch J (2006) Effect of rosiglitazone on the frequency of diabetes in patients with impaired glucose tolerance on impaired fasting glucose: a randomised controlled trial. *Lancet*, 368: 1096–105

Hansson L *et al.* (1998) The Hypertension Optimal Treatment (HOT) Study: 24 month data on blood pressure and tolerability. *Lancet* 351: 1755–612

HMSO (1999) *Saving Lives: Our Healthier Nation*. White Paper, Cm 4386. London: The Stationery Office

Marks L (1996) *Counting the Cost: The real impact of non-insulin dependent diabetes*. London: King's Fund/BDA

Medical Research Council/British Heart Foundation (2003) Heart Protection Study of cholesterol-lowering with simvastatin in 5963 individuals with diabetes: a randomised placebo-controlled trial. Heart Protection Study Collaborative Group. *Lancet* 361: 2005–16

Pierce M, Agarwal G, Ridout D (2000) A survey of diabetes care in general practice in England and Wales. *British Journal of General Practice* 50: 542–5

Royal College of Physicians/British Diabetic Association (1993) *Good Practice in the Diagnosis and Treatment of NIDDM*. London: RCP/BDA

UKPDS 33. *Lancet* 1998; 352: 837–53. UKPDS 36. *BMJ* 2000; 321: 412–19.

UKPDS 34. *Lancet* 1998; 352: 854–65. UKPDS 38. *BMJ* 1998; 317: 703–13.

UKPDS 35. *BMJ* 2000; 321: 405–12. UKPDS 39. *BMJ* 1998; 317: 713–20.

Books for health professionals

Dornhorst D, Hadden DR (eds) (1996) *Diabetes and Pregnancy: An international approach to diagnosis and management*. Chichester: John Wiley & Sons

Edmonds ME, Foster AVM (2005) *Managing the Diabetic Foot*, 2nd edn. Oxford: Blackwell Science

Foster MC, Cole M (1996) *Impotence: A guide to management*. London: Martin Dunitz

Hall, G (2007) *Providing Diabetes Care in General Practice: A practical guide for the primary care team*, 5th edn. London: Class Publishing

Taylor R (2006) *Handbook of Retinal Screening in Diabetes*. Chichester: John Wiley

Williams G, Pickup J (2004) *Handbook of Diabetes*, 3rd edn. Oxford: Blackwell Science

Books for patients

Campbell IW, Lebovitz H (1996) *Fast Facts – Diabetes Mellitus*. Oxford: Health Press

Day J (2001) *Living with Diabetes: the Diabetes UK guide for those treated with diet and tablets*. Chichester: John Wiley

Day J (2002) *Living with Diabetes: the Diabetes UK guide for those treated with insulin*. Chichester: John Wiley

Fahey T, Murphy D, Tudor Hart J (2004). *High Blood Pressure at Your Fingertips*, 3rd edn. London: Class Publishing

Fox C, Hanas R (2007) *Type 2 Diabetes in Adults of All Ages*. London: Class Publishing

Fox C, Kilvert A (2007) *Type 1 Diabetes: Answers at your fingertips*. London: Class Publishing

Fox C, Kilvert A (2007) *Type 2 Diabetes: Answers at your fingertips*. London: Class Publishing

Hanas R (2007) *Type 1 Diabetes in Children, Adolescents and Young Adults*, 3rd edn. London: Class Publishing

Hanas R, Fox C (2007) *Type 2 Diabetes*. London: Class Publishing

Stein A, Wild J (2007) *Kidney Failure Explained*, 3rd edn. London: Class Publishing

Walker R, Rodgers J (2004) *Diabetes: A practical guide to managing your health*. London: Dorling Kindersley

Multimedia

Learning Diabetes (insulin treated) and *Learning Diabetes (non-insulin treated)*
Multimedia patient education programmes produced as a package called Managing Your Health by Interactive Eurohealth. For information, please telephone or fax 01394 412141, or email sales@interactiveeurohealth.com

Journals

The Diabetic Foot
SB Communications Group*
Four issues per year

Diabetic Medicine
Issued 12 times per year
Can be purchased through professional membership sections of Diabetes UK

Diabetes and Primary Care
SB Communications Group*
Four issues per year

Diabetes Update
Periodic newsletter (free) for healthcare professionals interested in diabetes; available for Diabetes UK members

Journal of Diabetes Nursing
SB Communications Group*
Six issues per year

Practical Diabetes International
Nine issues per year, available from John Wiley & Sons**

* SB Communications Group, FREEPOST LON7814, London SE26 5BR

** John Wiley & Sons, 1 Oldlands Way, Bognor Regis, West Sussex PO22 9SA

KEY WEBSITES

Anglo-Scandinavian Cardiac Outcomes Trial (ASCOT) Full information on results and publications can be found on the study website: www.ascotstudy.org

DAFNE (Dose Adjustment For Normal Eating) – background to the study and follow-up information www.dafne.uk.com

Diabetes UK: www.diabetes.org.uk – first port of call for diabetes information on the Internet (for professionals and for patients/families)

Joslin Diabetes Centre – educational website: www.joslin.harvard.edu/education

Medscape – an excellent free resource with a section on diabetes: www.medscape.com

MRC/BHF Heart Protection Study – www.ctsu.ox.ac.uk/~hps/

Research and Development Learning database: www.rdlearning.org.uk – the best database for finding out what courses are available throughout the UK

Warwick Diabetes Care: www.diabetescare.warwick.ac.uk

The following provide drugs, equipment, booklets, leaflets, posters, videos, identification cards, monitoring diaries, GP information training, clinic packs, etc. (local representatives will have specific details of what is available). Please contact them at the telephone numbers given to find out exactly what they do provide.

Diabetes UK
10 Parkway
London NW1 7AA
Tel: 020 7424 1000
Fax: 020 7424 1001
Email: info@diabetes.org.uk
Website: www.diabetes.org.uk
Diabetes UK is the national organisation for people with diabetes. It is a very useful first point of contact for both professionals and patients for all sorts of information and advice from welfare benefits to holidays.
A publications list is available free from Diabetes UK: 0800 585088 (publications line). Some, but not all, titles are free. The most widely used titles are: *Food Choices and Diabetes*; *Treating your Diabetes with Tablets*; *Coping with Diabetes*; *When you are Ill*; *Diabetes: What care to expect*
For specific cultural information, please ring the Health Care Delivery Department at Diabetes UK
Tel: 020 7323 1531
Fax: 020 7637 3644

3M United Kingdom plc
Tel: 08705 360036

Aventis Pharma UK
Tel: 01732 584000
Fax: 01732 584080

Bayer plc
Tel: 01635 563000
Fax: 01635 566260
Helpline: 01635 566366

Becton Dickinson UK Ltd
Tel: 01865 748844
Fax: 01865 717313

Britannia Health Products
Tel: 01737 773741
Fax: 01737 779544

CP Pharmaceuticals
Tel: 01978 661261
Fax: 01978 660130

DVLA
(Drivers and Vehicles Licensing Authority)
Drivers Medical Group
Swansea
SA99 1DL
Tel: 0870 240 0009
Fax: 01792 761100

Golden Key Company
(SOS/Talisman)
Tel: 01795 663403
Fax: 01795 661356

GlaxoSmithKline
Tel: 020 8990 9000
Fax: 020 8990 4321

Hypoguard UK Ltd
Tel: 01394 387333/4
Fax: 01394 380152

LifeScan
Tel: 01494 450423
Fax: 01494 685751
Customer Careline: 0800 121200

Lilly Diabetes Care Division
Tel: 01256 315000

Medic-Alert Foundation
British Isles & Ireland
Tel: 020 7833 3034
Fax: 020 7278 0647
Helpline: 0800 581420

Merck Pharmaceuticals Ltd
Tel: 01895 452200
Fax: 01895 452274

Novo Nordisk UK
Tel: 01293 613555
Fax: 01293 613535
Customer Careline: 0845 6005055

Owen Mumford Ltd
Tel: 01993 812021
Fax: 01993 813466

Pfizer
Tel: 01304 616161
Fax: 01304 656221

Pharmacia Ltd
Tel: 01670 562400
Fax: 01670 562401

Quitline
(For help in stopping smoking)
Tel: 0800 002200

Roche Diagnostics
Tel: 01273 480444
Fax: 01273 480266
Direct Order Line: 0800 701000

Servier Laboratories Ltd
Tel: 01753 662744
Fax: 01753 663456

Smith & Nephew
Health Care Ltd
Tel: 01482 222200
Fax: 01482 222211
Helpline: 0800 590173

INSURANCES, FINANCE AND PENSIONS

Diabetes UK Services
Term Assurance Quoteline
Insurance Advice Line
and Financial Services
Tel: 0800 731 7431

Devitt Insurance
Services Ltd
Tel: 01708 385959
Fax: 0870 241 2358

Feedback Form

We, the authors, would welcome your comments on this book. Would you like more on some subjects and less on others? Are there additional topics which you would like to see in future editions? Please help us by marking your comments on this page, and sending it to the publisher, post-free, at

Class Publishing, FREEPOST, London, W6 7BR

Current topics

	More?	Less?
1 The impact of living with diabetes	☐	☐
2 Insights into type 2 diabetes	☐	☐
3 National Service Frameworks and NICE	☐	☐
4 Screening and identification	☐	☐
5 Early management of type 2 diabetes	☐	☐
6 Educating patients about managing type 2 diabetes	☐	☐
7 Longer term management of type 2 diabetes	☐	☐
8 How to control blood glucose levels	☐	☐
9 How to reduce long-term complications of diabetes	☐	☐
10 How to manage type 1 diabetes	☐	☐
11 How to manage pregnancy and gestational diabetes	☐	☐
12 Living with diabetes	☐	☐
13 Emergencies and illness	☐	☐
14 Diabetes care and general practice	☐	☐

Additional topics

....

....

....

Other comments

....

....

....

May we contact you?

NAME

OCCUPATION

ADDRESS

TOWN   POSTCODE

*Have you found **Vital Diabetes** useful and practical? If so, you may be interested in these other books on from Class Publishing.*

NEW!

Providing Diabetes Care in General Practice £29.99

Gwen Hall

Mary MacKinnon's classic textbook for the Practice Diabetes Team has been completely revised and updated by one of the leading names in diabetes care today. Maintaining the breadth, vision and authority of the original, this new edition takes into account recent developments in service structure and healthcare policy, research, education and much, much more.

> *'Gwen Hall is to be congratulated in retaining the spirit of the original, but imbuing it with her own personality. The best just got better. Treasure it.'*

> **Dr Eugene Hughes**, Chairman, Primary Care Diabetes Europe

COMING SOON!

Type 1 Diabetes: Answers at your fingertips £14.99

Type 2 Diabetes: Answers at your fingertips £14.99

Both by Dr Charles Fox and Dr Anne Kilvert

For your patients, and for you.
The latest edition of our bestselling reference guide on diabetes has now been split into two books covering the two distinct forms of the disease. These books maintain the popular question and answer format to provide practical advice for patients on every aspect of living with the condition. *Available mid 2007*

Chronic Obstructive Pulmonary Disease in Primary Care £29.99

Dr David Bellamy and Rachel Booker

This clear and helpful resource manual addresses the management requirements of GPs and practice nurses. In this book, you will find guidance, protocols, plans and tests – all appropriate to the primary care situation – that will streamline your diagnosis and management of COPD.

> *'I am sure it will become a classic in the history of COPD Care.'*

> **Duncan Geddes**, Professor of Respiratory Medicine and Consultant Physician, Royal Brompton Hospital

Heart Health: Answers at your fingertips £14.99

Dr Graham Jackson

This practical handbook, written by a leading cardiologist, answers many of your patients' questions about heart conditions. It gives the reader information about their own health and their heart; how to keep the heart healthy, or – if it has been affected by heart disease – how to make it as strong as possible.

> *'Those readers who want to know more about the various treatments for heart disease will be much enlightened.'*

> **Dr James Le Fanu**, *The Daily Telegraph*

VITAL BOOKS FOR YOUR PRACTICE TEAM

The definitive quick reference manuals for all health professionals

Armed with these straightforward handbooks, you can treat patients with speed and confidence. Ideal for GPs, practice nurses, specialist nurses, community pharmacists and students.

VITAL ASTHMA

Sue Cross and Dave Burns

VITAL NEPHROLOGY

Dr Andy Stein, Janet Wild and Dr Paul Cook

VITAL COPD

Rachel Booker

VITAL LUNG FUNCTION

Rachel Booker

This series provides you with:

- Clear and concise information at a glance

- All the essential medical background you need for daily practice

- Patient information sections to help you explain complex subjects

- 'Vital Points' highlighted throughout the text for easy reference

- Up-to-date information to help you structure treatment in primary care

Priority Order Form

Cut out or photocopy this form and send it (post-free in the UK) to:

**Class Publishing, FREEPOST 16705, Macmillan Distribution, Basingstoke RG21 6ZZ
Tel: 01256 302 699 / Fax: 01256 812 558**

Please send me urgently

No. of copies		Post included price per copy (UK only)
_____	*Vital Diabetes* (ISBN 10:1 85959 174 4 / ISBN 13:978 1 85959 174 1)	£17.99
_____	*Vital Asthma* (ISBN 10:1 85959 107 8 / ISBN 13:978 1 85959 107 9)	£17.99
_____	*Vital Nephrology* (ISBN 10:1 85959 102 7 / ISBN 13:978 1 85959 102 4)	£17.99
_____	*Vital COPD* (ISBN 10:1 85959 114 0 / ISBN 13:978 1 85959 114 7)	£17.99
_____	*Vital Lung Function* (ISBN 10:1 85959 161 2 / ISBN 13:978 1 85959 161 1)	£17.99
_____	*Providing Diabetes Care in General Practice* (ISBN 10:1 85959 154 X / ISBN 13:978 1 85959 154 3)	£32.99
_____	*COPD in Primary Care* (ISBN 10:1 85959 104 3 / ISBN 13:978 1 85959 140 8)	£32.99
_____	*Type 1 Diabetes – Answers at your fingertips* (ISBN 10:1 85959 175 2 / ISBN 13:978 1 85959 175 8)	£17.99
_____	*Type 2 Diabetes – Answers at your fingertips* (ISBN 10:1 85959 176 0 / ISBN 13:978 1 85959 176 5)	£17.99
_____	*Heart Health – Answers at your fingertips* (ISBN 10:1 85959 157 4 / ISBN 13:978 1 85959 157 4)	£17.99

TOTAL   £_____

Easy ways to pay

1. *I enclose a cheque made payable to Class Publishing for* £_____

2. *Please charge my*   Mastercard ☐   Visa ☐   Amex ☐

CARD NUMBER   EXPIRY DATE

NAME

MY ADDRESS FOR DELIVERY IS

TOWN   COUNTY   POSTCODE

TELEPHONE NUMBER (*in case of query*)

CREDIT CARD BILLING ADDRESS (*if different from above*)

TOWN   COUNTY   POSTCODE

Class Publishing's guarantee: remember that if, for any reason, you are not satisfied with these books, we will refund all your money, without any questions asked. Prices and VAT rates may be altered for reasons beyond our control.